HOW TO LOSE WEIGHT IN THE REAL WORLD

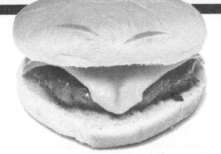

Why Other Diets Suck and You're Not Losing Weight

Dr. J. deValentino

First Edition

Houston, Texas

How to Lose Weight in the Real World
Why Other Diets Suck and You're Not Losing Weight by Dr. J. deValentino

DeValentino Publishing
P.O. Box 420613
Houston, Texas 77242
j@devalentino.com; www.devalentino.com

Unattributed quotes are by Dr. J. deValentino

ISBN: 978-0-9828946-0-6

Library of Congress Cataloging-in-Publication Data

deValentino, Jessica
   How to lose weight in the real world : why other diets suck and you're not losing
      weight / by Jessica deValentino
   Includes bibliographical references and index.
ISBN-13: 978-0-9828946-0-6
      1. Nutrition—United States I. deValentino, Jessica. How to lose weight in the
real world: why other diets suck and you're not losing weight

Contents

Dedication

To Jesse Howe, my grandfather.

I wish I knew what I know a lot sooner to share with you.

Dear Reader,

While this book attempts to holistically address dietary information, relevant and new information may have been overlooked. Please feel free to e-mail me at *j@devalentino.com* to address any issues, which will be taken into consideration for the next edition.

> *"The way to keep your health is to eat what you don't want, drink what you don't like, and do what you'd rather not."*
> — MARK TWAIN (1835–1910) U.S. HUMORIST, WRITER, AND LECTURER.

Dear reader, please excuse the error in the vegetarian stars table on page 77; it should read:
Flexibility ★★★
Health ★★★
Maintainability ★★★
Satisfaction ★★★

WARNING–DISCLAIMER

ATTENTION: Educational institutions and industry publications: Quantity discounts are available on bulk purchases of this book for reselling, educational purposes, gifts, or fund raisers. Modifications of this book can be created to fit specific needs. For information, please send an inquiry.

HOW TO CONTACT THE AUTHOR

Dr. deValentino is a faculty member at the University of Phoenix and professional speaker. Dr. deValentino is delighted to enrich and inform audiences regarding social constructs. To discuss hiring her for your next conference, fundraiser, or special event, contact:

> Dr. Jessica deValentino
> P.O. Box 420613, Houston, Texas 77242
> www.devalentino.com / j@devalentino.com
> 713.530.5505

Part I

What You Need to Know

What You Don't Know Can Hurt You

"When we know better, we do better."
— MAYA ANGELOU

THE MERE MENTION OF the word "diet" can dredge up horrific memories of yucky concoctions, bland food, and starvation. There are so many diets available, which is right? Which one is going to work? The meat diet, the soda diet, the sugar diet, or the cookie diet? None of the above. You don't have to go on some weird, distressing diet to lose weight. Forget about the strictly regimented, no calorie, low carb, special drink, eat only on the prime dates, but not while the sun is shining, non-deviation plan diets.

Food is a non-negotiable, it is a part of life and it shouldn't be avoided. Food is the center of entertainment, rewards, punishment, celebrations, mourning, and numerous other occasions. With a date comes dinner out, with parties come hors d'oeuvres, with a birthday comes... you guessed it, cake. There are so many restaurants and advertisers working feverishly to break our resistance. Being constantly bombarded with food that looks good and tastes even better is troublesome for the best of folks. We've all happily indulged in food on more than one occasion.

You are not alone in the struggle to lose weight and keep it off. Currently in United States there are approximately 200 million people battling to win the war of the pounds, and statistics report that over 95% of people who lose weight will regain it, which also means many people try unsuccessful diets and weight loss plans that don't result in permanent weight loss.

Food is a double-edged sword; it can keep you alive, but it can also kill you. Food's purpose as nourishment has become convoluted and distorted by the desire to indulge the taste buds, increase convenience, and reduce costs; but it doesn't have to be the nemesis. While food does satisfy your indulgences, it also provides energy and nutrients. There are a lot of factors contending on what foods you eat such as advertising, convenience, location, preferences, and time. So what wins out in the end?

There are many reasons to put off eating right. Yes, there are the arguments like, "Life is short. Everyone dies. Live it up and be happy. Eating right can start tomorrow. Healthy food isn't real food, it's rabbit food. Healthy food just doesn't taste good. Tomorrow isn't promised." Those arguments may be true, but they are not a good reason for you to sabotage your health. Your body carries you through time; do all that you can to maintain your time machine. Hasty decisions may slide today; however, they may destroy your health years later, so give your future a fighting chance. Changes later may be too late.

Somewhere inside of you, you want to do better. Small modifications will help you live better and enjoy your life infinitely more while possibly avoiding painful, agonizing, and crippling results of poor health maintenance. By taking care of yourself, you may reduce the cost and time associated with treating various health complications.

Many people have erroneously attributed lifestyle choices to genetics, believing that they are destined to endure a dismal fate because of genetics; however, scientific studies are proving otherwise. There are environmental factors that may have a more profound effect on your health than genetics. Environmental factors include eating habits, lifestyle, and external conditions; factors that you can actually manage.

Research studies have found that environmental factors, such as your diet, show a stronger correlation to obesity than genetics. Even animals of weight-challenged individuals have been found to be overweight. Many people love their animals, but they did not birth them. Don't let genetics stop you from losing weight—you determine your fate, not your family's history. So that age-old excuse "I am weight-challenged because my momma, grandpa, auntie, cousin, brother, are too," may be out the window.

So what really happens when families and animals share weight issues? Many of us are creatures of habit. Throughout life our cultures, eating styles, habits, and preferences become engrained in us. After living and eating with our families for about two decades, their way of life is bound to influence our decisions. Therefore, before you jump to the conclusion that there is no way around predisposed genetic factors, take your destiny into your hands and create your fate.

The same goes for devastating illnesses like cancer. A group of scientists have estimated that genetics only accounts for 2–3% of the risk for getting many diseases, and that a significant portion of the risk is attributable to diet and lifestyle, as evidenced through animal experimentations that resulted in increased and decreased cancer growth with diet manipulation.

Although genetics may have an effect on health, it is not the ultimate power; you have the ability to positively impact your health. Genes have the ability to be turned off or on like switch. Researchers have found that environmental factors can turn on previously dormant conditions. Taking care of yourself is a good way to keep bad genes inactive.

Many of us look forward to the next opportunity to eat—where will we eat, what will we eat, how much will we eat; but instead of satisfying our desire to eat, we have to stop and evaluate our food. When we make poor dietary decisions, it is usually based on information that we had collected over time that influence our decisions—like fat is bad, eat low carbs; don't eat too much salt, chicken and pasta dishes are healthy diet dishes, protein bars are good, and anything with wheat on the label is nutritious. Tons of suggestions and advice swirl around in our minds, clouding our judgment.

One of the most significant contributing factors to the steady increase of weight since the 1960s in the US is the sheer quantity of confusing and erroneous information presented as the sure-fire way to lose weight. There is an urgent need to holistically improve dietary knowledge in the US. Flawed information keeps people making poor dietary decisions that have significant future health ramifications.

We are constantly assaulted with snippets of health and diet information from family, friends, the Internet, magazines, news, radio, and talk shows that present out of context information as the gospel. The conflicting dietary information about what to eat and what not to eat muddles an already jumbled picture. Random recommendations without solid rationales are difficult for nearly everyone to follow successfully. In order to make better decisions you must fully understand the effect of food on not only your diet, but your health.

Holistic information will help you make better food-related decisions to improve your weight and health. Knowing how food affects your body will help change the way that you think about food and the way you eat. Losing weight requires a conscious, educated decision about every morsel that enters your mouth. Learning about your diet will help you intuitively select healthier foods while reducing and eliminating foods that are adverse to improving your health and decreasing your weight. Knowledge is the tool to help you make better decisions to help you reach your weight goals and make it easy to eat anywhere from home, to restaurants, to parties.

After reading this information you will be able to navigate through oceans of incalculable food choices. This book will reveal the hidden dangers and nuances of food to help you improve your health and weight. As many as 63% of Americans report they are confused by all of the conflicting nutritional information. If you are a member of this group, sit back, relax, and continue reading to help your confusion become a thing of the past.

What Food Can Do to Your Body 2

"An ounce of prevention is worth more than a pound of cure."
— UNKNOWN

LOSING WEIGHT IS NOT the only reason to make dietary enhancements. Improving your diet can be beneficial to not only your weight, but your health by reducing the risk of disease and illness, while improving the appearance of your hair, nails, and skin, and increasing your level of energy.

Over the last twenty years, the obesity rates in the United States have skyrocketed. Obesity does not discriminate against age, education level, ethnicity, geographic region, race, sex, or socioeconomic status. Obesity rates among adults have doubled, while obesity rates among children 6–19 years old have quadrupled to approximately 16%. According to National Health and Nutrition Examination Survey (NHANES, 2004) approximately two-thirds or 133 million adults are overweight while approximately one-third or 66 million adults are obese.

Overweight and obese are recognized as the accumulation of excess body fat that may have negative effects on health and will likely reduce life expectancy. BMI stands for Body Mass Index and it is a way to quickly and easily identify overweight and obese individuals based on height and weight. Overweight is differentiated by having a BMI of 23.0 to 24.9, whereas obese is designated by BMI over 25. BMI disregards several important factors such as age, gender, and muscle content, which can significantly skew the results. For instance, muscular individuals may fall into the "overweight" category, when actually they may be quite fit.

There are many negative outcomes associated with obesity including arthritis, diabetes, heart disease, high blood pressure, and multiple forms of cancer. The annual health care cost attributed to treating obesity and obesity-related illness is estimated to be over $240 billion and an additional $33 billion on diet and weight loss plans. Obesity creates many health related concerns, consequences, and complications including, but not limited to:

+ Stroke
+ Osteoarthritis
+ Increased mortality
+ Stress incontinence
+ Increased surgical risk
+ Liver and gallbladder disease
+ Complications with pregnancy
+ Sleep apnea and respiratory problems
+ Psychological disorders like depression
+ Hirsutism (presence of excess body and facial hair)
+ Dyslipidemia (high total cholesterol or triglycerides)
+ Gynecological problems (abnormal menses and infertility)
  (NIDDK, 2008)

Research studies show that epic increases in cancer and degenerative diseases are significantly correlated to poor nutrition. As the American diet continues to deteriorate, the rate of disease continues to increase. Diet has an immense effect on health. Epidemiologists report that 35% of cancer can be attributed to the consumption of a poor diet. Although the cause of cancer is not definitive, many of the identified causal factors are manageable like alcohol, diet, lack of exercise, occupation, smoking, and sunning.

A poor diet facilitates the development of disease and illness, which may result in symptoms like allergies, back pain, bad breath, body odor, constipation, excess body weight, fatigue, gastrointestinal problems, reproduction complications, and skin disorders. Continued poor nutrition may develop into more serious problems like autoimmune diseases, cancer, compromised immune system, depressed metabolism, enzyme dysfunctions, hormonal imbalances, nutritional deficiencies, and toxin overload. Although some people may want to attribute the increase in health complications to old age or genetics, high consumption of inflammatory foods devoid of nutritional value is a real problem.

Eating habits have the ability to greatly influence the health of individuals. Therefore, every consideration should be given to what you eat daily. Making positive changes in your diet can provide immense savings to your medical expenses and your life. Chronic diseases take years to develop. In the meantime, much can to be done to reduce the likelihood of developing diseases by learning what modifications to make. The body has an amazing ability to heal itself when given the right ingredients.

Free Radicals

"All bodies are slow in growth but rapid in decay."
— PUBLIUS CORNELIUS TACITUS (55–117), ROMAN HISTORIAN.

Free radicals exist throughout the body and the environment. Free radicals are generated through normal metabolic processes, but there are also external sources of free radicals that attack the body that are found in air pollutants, alcohol, anesthetics, chemotherapy, cigarette smoke, formaldehyde, fried food, hydrocarbons, ionized radiation, pesticides, and solvents.

Free radicals may be formed in a reaction to a variety of elements including, but not limited to: metabolic activity, pollutants, and radiation. When this happens, molecular bonds weaken to form highly unstable molecules seeking electrons to become stable. Stealing electrons from another source damages the body and creates more free radicals. Free radicals attack and mutate DNA, which leads to the development of cancer. Aging appears to occur faster in some individuals than others, which may be associated with excessive free radicals.

The body can neutralize the mayhem caused by free radicals by utilizing the antioxidants within fruits and vegetables. Antioxidants are extremely helpful in maintaining the well-being of the body. During oxidation, free radicals are prepped to wreak havoc throughout the body until antioxidants come to the rescue. When antioxidants are not available, free radicals bond to parts within the body, which causes damage. Antioxidants protect against free radicals and carcinogens. Antioxidants neutralize the negative effect of the free radicals, thereby ending their reign of destruction.

Antioxidants are naturally found in plants. Although antioxidants are available in the form of vitamin supplements, recent studies have shown that consuming extra synthetic antioxidants does not provide any significant health benefits. The most benefits can be obtained from natural unrefined fruits and vegetables.

Inflammation

External inflammation is generally recognized as a tender, red, swollen, pain, stricken area of the body, but internal inflammation is not as easily recognizable. Internal inflammation is a symptomless complication that may not be seen or felt that damages DNA, hardens the arteries, facilitates the development of disease, increases the likelihood of a stroke and heart disease, increases the risk of infections, promotes cancer, and accelerates the aging process.

Normal cell functions, as well as environmental toxins, create free radicals that cause internal inflammation throughout the body. Inflammation is exacerbated by excess body fat, excessive unmanaged stress, insufficient exercise, sugar, toxins, and unhealthy diets.

The typical American diet contains insufficient anti-inflammatory foods and mega amounts of pro-inflammatory foods that debilitate and weaken the body. Research studies show that fast food meals create more free radicals than meals of fresh fruits, healthy fats, proteins, and vegetables. Pro-inflammatory conditions are promoted by:

+ Cooking oils
+ Excess weight
+ Deep-fried foods
+ Pre-packaged foods
+ Anti-inflammatory drugs
+ Insufficient fruits and vegetables

Although inflammation is common, chronic inflammation is a sign of serious health problems that weaken the body. Inflammation can delay healing, while chronic inflammation taxes the body and leads to disease. Many researchers believe that chronic inflammation within the body may lead to the development of autoimmune diseases and cancer. Food is not the only cause of inflammation; conditions that promote chronic inflammation within the body include:

+ Physical injuries
+ Frequent infections
+ Age-related atrophy
+ Allergies (food, intolerances, mold, pollen, etc.)
+ Environmental stress (radiation, smoke, sun, toxins)

Millions of Americans suffer from numerous inflammation disorders. The suffix "itis" identifies many inflammatory diseases. For example:

+ Hepatitis—inflammation of the liver
+ Arthritis—inflammation of the joints
+ Dermatitis—inflammation of the skin
+ Nephritis—inflammation of the kidney
+ Diverticulitis—inflammation of the intestinal wall
+ Colitis—inflammation of the colon or large intestine

Each year inflammation sufferers seek relief in the form of 30 billion over-the-counter non-steroidal anti-inflammatory drugs (NSAIDs), with an additional 70 million stronger varieties of NSAIDs prescribed by physicians. Excessive use of NSAIDs can cause ulcers and internal bleeding.

Environmental and chemical toxins continuously attack the body; the best way to detoxify the body is not by eliminating food, but rather eating foods high in natural enzymes and antioxidants that will reduce inflammation. Fiber is especially important in reducing levels of toxins in the body because it has the ability to absorb and expel them.

Eating anti-inflammatory foods is crucial to reducing inflammation inside of the body and losing weight. Inflammation reduces the resources available to heal the body. There are a wide variety of foods that can help eliminate inflammation and restore health to the body, which include eggs, fish, freshly squeezed juices (not the concentrate or bottled variety that have limited nutrients), fruits, herbs, nuts, omega-3 fatty acids, seeds (not salted or roasted), spices, teas, vegetables, and yogurt.

Flavonoids are a form of antioxidants produced by plants. Flavonoids are very beneficial to the human body; they have the ability to guard against allergies, cancer, inflammation, oxidants, and viruses. More than 5,000 flavonoids have been identified, so there are many opportunities to incorporate them into your diet.

Allergies and More

There are two main types of food sensitivities—food allergies and food intolerances. The Food Allergy and Anaphylaxis Network (FAAN) reports that over 11 million Americans are hypersensitive to some foods known as food allergens. As children age, sometimes they overcome allergies.

The body's immune system is designed to provide protection from invaders, and unfortunately some foods are seen as invaders, which triggers the body's attack mode. Allergens can be particularly tough on the immune system. Allergens can promote inflammation within the body, reduce the body's ability to operate efficiently and effectively, and thereby may increase body weight by promoting water retention, which causes swelling and bloating.

Unknown food allergens may significantly impact health and impede weight loss. The body may have an immediate or delayed response to allergens. Allergens initiate a series of reactions in the body that upset natural bodily functions. It is important to identify and eliminate any allergens in your diet to help your body perform optimally.

Approximately 140 food allergens have been identified; however, according to the Center for Disease Control, 90% of all allergies are attributed to eight categories of food allergens. Even small amounts of allergens may evoke an allergic reaction. The eight categories of food allergens include:

+ Milk
+ Eggs
+ Wheat
+ Peanuts
+ Soybeans
+ Fish (cod, haddock, halibut, herring, mackerel, and trout)
+ Shellfish (crab, crustaceans, lobster, prawns, shellfish, and shrimp)

✦ Tree nuts (almonds, brazil nuts, cashews, chestnuts, hazelnuts, pecans, pistachios, and walnuts)

Food allergies may cause a series of symptoms including:
✦ Hives
✦ Nausea
✦ Rashes
✦ Itching
✦ Asthma
✦ Fainting
✦ Diarrhea
✦ Sneezing
✦ Headaches
✦ Swelling of body parts
✦ Breathing complications

People with multiple allergies may wonder what foods will not promote an allergic response. Non-allergenic foods include, but are not limited to:
✦ Rice
✦ Pears
✦ Lamb
✦ Apples
✦ Carrots
✦ Cherries
✦ Sesame Seeds
✦ Winter Squash
✦ Sweet Potatoes

Food is not the only source of allergens; environmental allergens can significantly impact the body as well. Environmental allergens may include dust, mold, pollen, and toxins, all of which may promote inflammation within the body.

Not all negative reactions are triggered by food allergies; some are caused by varying degrees of sensitivity to food known as food intolerances. A food intolerance is a reproducible negative response, which unlike a food allergy, does not involve an autoimmune response. Some of the main foods associated with food intolerances include, but are not limited to, food additives, gluten, lactose, preservatives, and tyrosine. While allergic reactions may be full-blown within minutes, food intolerances may fester and manifest 24 to 48 hours later, making it difficult to identify the offending culprit. Food intolerances may cause the same problems as food allergies, but also may cause bloating, eating disorders, fatigue, gas, migraines, mood swings, and nervousness.

Elimination diets help identify the source of food allergies and intolerances. Elimination diets can be easily initiated by eliminating one of the major allergy offenders from your diet at a time for a week or two. During the elimination period, it is important to take detailed notes of any differences that you notice with your body and health. If you identify the culprit, great! If not, it's back to the drawing board, eliminating another one of the eight common food allergens or a food that you suspect may be causing problems while still evaluating the differences that you observe in your health and body. In some cases, it may be a combination of foods that produce ill effects, so it is important not to reintroduce previously eliminated foods until all of the offending culprits have been identified. When you finally decide to reintroduce eliminated foods into your diet, carefully assess your overall condition. If you do not arrive at any solid answers, a doctor may be able to identify the allergen from the antibodies present in your blood sample.

Metabolic Syndrome

Metabolic syndrome or insulin resistance syndrome affects roughly 50 to 100 million Americans and is known as a group of symptoms that increases the likelihood of developing diabetes, heart attack, or stroke. Metabolic syndrome can be improved with a healthy diet. The factors that contribute to metabolic syndrome include:

+ Inflammation
+ Insulin resistance—body's resistance to insulin
+ High blood pressure—130/85 mm hg or higher
+ Prothrombotic condition—increased likelihood for blood clots
+ Excess abdominal fat; for men a waist $\geq$ 40; for women a waist $\geq$ 35
+ Hyperlipidemia—high levels of triglycerides and lipids (fats) in the blood

Diabetes

Diabetes develops when the body cannot properly reduce blood sugar levels after eating. High blood sugar levels negatively impact the body. Over time, elevated blood sugar may cause a series of problems like diabetes, insulin resistance, metabolic syndrome, and obesity. Diabetes has steadily increased over the last century to unprecedented rates. In the US there are approximately 24 million people with diabetes and more than 100 billion dollars is spent every year to help them live with the disease.

Diabetes contributes to a series of health complications such as amputations, blindness, cancer, cardiovascular disease, dental disease, high blood pressure, kidney disease, nerve degeneration in the legs, pregnancy complications, stroke, and death.

There are two types of diabetes. Type I diabetes generally occurs early in life and is sometimes known as juvenile diabetes. Type I diabetes occurs in 5–10% of diabetes cases. With type I diabetes the pancreas does not manufacture and secrete enough insulin, leaving high levels of glucose in the blood. External sources of insulin are required to regulate blood glucose levels.

The majority of diabetics, 90–95%, have type II diabetes. Type II diabetes occurs during adulthood and is also known adult-onset diabetes. However, with poor diet regimens type II diabetes is becoming more prevalent in children; therefore, the age-specific names are being retired. Researchers have found that excess weight significantly increases the risks of individuals contracting diabetes. With type II diabetes, the pancreas produces insulin; however, due to excessive weight and poor diet, the body is not able to sufficiently reduce blood glucose levels. Unhealthy diets and body fat reduce the effectiveness of insulin, and as a result the body require extra external sources of insulin to effectively regulate blood sugar. Body fat makes cells resistant to insulin. Although insulin regulates blood glucose levels, it also promotes weight gain and exacerbates diabetes. Excess weight and body fat reduce the effectiveness of insulin, thus requiring more and more insulin and creating a vicious cycle. Fats, fibers, and proteins slow the absorption of sugars into the blood. Lemon juice and vinegar help reduce blood sugar levels as much as 30%.

Eight to 18% of diabetics are newly diagnosed with cancer. Researchers have found that people with diabetes are more likely to die of cancer due to high blood sugar levels that nourish cancer and promote tumor growth. Diabetes-related problems may make it difficult to diagnose the presence of cancer until the later stages, thus limiting treatment options, increasing susceptibility to infection, and preventing aggressive treatment due to the body's weakened state.

Studies show that there is a relationship between diabetes and cardiac disease. The likelihood of experiencing a heart attack increases 400% for diabetics versus non-diabetics while studies have shown that 70% of all individuals with diabetes will die from a heart attack or stroke.

The good news is that diabetes can generally be controlled, even eliminated, with a good diet. Research studies confirm a reduction in nutrient-deficient food and an increase in unrefined and unprocessed carbohydrates may significantly control blood sugar enough to eliminate medication.

Heart Disease

In the US, the number one killer, even more deadly than diabetes and cancer, is heart disease. Heart attacks strike almost 1.5 million people each year and 500,000 do not survive, claiming over 30% of all deaths each year. Upon the untimely death of many healthy young men, women, and children, autopsies reveal the development of heart disease. Without the necessary dietary improvements, heart disease will claim the life of one in three Americans.

Heart disease can be prevented and even reversed with adequate precautions; however, each year in the US approximately 400,000 heart surgeries offer a life extension to people who realized they'd do anything to live, which includes having their chest cracked open and veins sliced and re-routed for as much as $60,000. If cardiac patients make it out of the surgery alive, cause everyone doesn't, they're still not out of the woods yet. There are a series of maladies that wait such as bleeding complications, heart attack, high blood pressure, infection, respiratory complications, and stroke.

Although heart surgery may give a new lease on life, the lease is not permanent. In fact, studies show that plaque grows faster after surgery. Restenosis, a physician-generated disease, inhibits the body's ability to heal naturally. Unfortunately 70 to 80% of the heart bypass surgery patients may feel the excruciating heart pain again within three years while arteries treated by angioplasty may become clogged in four to six months.

Blood pressure medications reduce the occurrence of a heart attack; however, dietary changes are necessary to significantly reduce the likelihood of a fatal heart attack. A research study involving 20 countries shows that populations that consumed less saturated fat and meat while eating more fruit, vegetables, and whole grains, have less heart disease. Eating unhealthy foods deposits plaque, promotes blood clots, and stiffens veins and arteries. By eliminating or reducing bad oils, dairy, meats, and poultry, people have the opportunity to reverse the effects of heart disease and eliminate medication.

Alzheimer's Disease

Alzheimer's is a dreadful mind-debilitating disease that ultimately leaves the sufferer unable to recall familiar faces and do the simplest tasks. Some researchers are starting to believe that unhealthy food is at the root cause of Alzheimer's. Studies have shown that antioxidants provide protection to the body against physiological damage and free radicals and this protection extends to the brain. Just as good nutrition helps, poor nutrition hurts. Poor nutrition promotes the development of free radicals that exacerbate mental diseases. Research data shows that populations that consume less meat have fewer cases of Alzheimer's.

Most individuals affected by Alzheimer's disease also suffer from cardiovascular disease, stroke, and type II diabetes. Experimental animal studies show that high cholesterol levels contribute to beta-amyloid production, the key negative factor of Alzheimer's. Plus, individuals with low levels of folic acid, an element common in plant products, were more than three times likely to develop Alzheimer's.

Colorectal Cancer

The development of a cancerous growth in the colon, rectum, or appendix is known as colorectal cancer. Colorectal cancer is the fifth most common type of cancer in the US. Colorectal cancer generally begins as a benign polyp that develops into cancer over time. Early detection offers a good chance of a cure through surgery, chemotherapy, or radiation; however, left untreated, the cancer may spread throughout the body with a fatal outcome.

Although there are some unalterable risks factors like age, heredity, and history of cancer, there are still steps that you can take to reduce the likelihood of developing cancer like eat more fruits and vegetables, get a colonoscopy, limit meat, quit smoking, and reduce alcohol.

Another important factor in reducing the rate of contracting colorectal cancer is exercise. A series of research studies all conclude that exercise significantly reduces the risk of contracting colon cancer. This may be due to the increased circulation and stimulation of the bowel.

Conclusion

Although research shows that environmental factors are stronger predictors for health than genetics, it is important to cover all of your bases and take the necessary precautions to have the best life possible. Review your family's medical history; having a close relative with a medical condition or illness may increase the likelihood that you may develop the same condition. Visit your doctor yearly for exams and diagnostic treatments. Depending on your beliefs, this might be the only life you'll get.

Health problems do not happen overnight. Chronic diseases generally take years to develop. The advances in science have identified many lifestyle factors that promote the development of disease and how to reduce and eliminate the possibility of disease. You can improve your diet and health, or you can indifferently enjoy the goodies and pay the piper later. If you put in the effort now, there is a greater chance of success. If you don't take adequate precautions, then you may have to rely on others to restore your health. Let's check out the help that is available if we fall sick in the next chapter.

Who and What Can Help? 3

A T TIMES, the conflicting nutritional information from trusted sources may be confusing. Some sources have a vested interest in the confusion and diminished health of the general public. You may be wondering what anyone could have to gain from the deteriorating health of others? Illness is a big business, and it is not in the best interest of the food, medical, and pharmaceutical industries for people to suddenly realize the danger of poor nutrition.

Erroneous information is advertised everywhere. Why? Well, a lot is riding on what the public consumes daily. Money makes people do strange things, and with over a trillion dollars at stake between the food, medical, and pharmaceutical industries, it is understandable why 100% honesty is not the rule, but the exception.

So who is going to tell you everything you need to know? In order to get the best information, you must carefully analyze and gather information to make good decisions to protect your health. Equip yourself with the knowledge necessary to make good dietary decisions, despite the random recommendations and tidbits of information floating around.

There is a pinch of truth in the best lies. Many advertisers and food companies rely on reductionism, which takes the truth out of context. A purely hypothetical example: let's say the newest super food is pineapple. If you eat pineapple you'll grow stronger. The exact element in pineapple that promotes strength is not known, but enzyme z is one of the elements in pineapple; therefore, enzyme z may make you stronger. The food industry promotes pineapple as the new super fruit and everyone eats pineapples, but this cuts drug manufacturers out of the loop, but not for long, because if you think enzyme z will make you stronger the drug companies will most likely tell you that you can save yourself the time and trouble of eating pineapple and get enzyme z in a handy dandy little pill. The drug companies will not mention that natural unrefined pineapple, like all fruits, is a storehouse of nutrients and fiber and has countless benefits that are not available in the pill. Supplements only serve up limited and processed nutrients.

Many nutritionists argue that the recommendations from many trusted and reputable organizations do not support good health. The Department of Agriculture and Health and Human Services (USDA/HHS) have released multiple revisions of the Dietary Guidelines for Americans in 1985, 1990, 1995, 2000, 2005, and 2010. With each revision, there are multiple drafts to allow food and agriculture industries to ensure their economics are not damaged. The welfare of the industries is considered, but who is looking out for the welfare of the public? Recommendations from the food industry's special interest groups carry a lot of weight. In the past 10 years the food industry has spent approximately one billion dollars lobbying politicians. At one point, the Agriculture Department wanted the average daily diet to consist of 2,350 calories, mainly to ensure that large portions were not reduced; fortunately a 2,000 calorie diet was settled upon, which is still significantly more than most people need.

The RDAs are not always set with the best interest of individuals, but rather corporate industries. The sugar industry challenged the upper safe limits of sugar recommendations to ensure the public did not perceive the daily sugar requirements unsafe, and thereby decrease their profits. The RDA affects food labels and food available in hospitals; nursing homes; schools; the Women, Infants, and Children (WIC) program; and other government funded food programs. The most unfortunate effect of the RDA is on the school lunch program. Guidelines failing to take into account the dangers of too much fat and sugar in the daily diet, may establish poor eating habits and promote obesity in children.

Health Care

"The doctor is often more to be feared than the disease."
— FRENCH PROVERB

Many industrialized nations provide health care for all citizens; however, it is estimated that more than 45 million Americans do not have health insurance. A national survey reports that the primary reason for the uninsured is the high cost associated with health insurance. In 2007, 2.4 trillion dollars was spent on the health care industry, a number that greatly exceeds that of other countries due to administrative fees, fraud, mismanagement, and waste. But there is even more to fret about, because this number is expected to skyrocket in the near future.

Illness puts people at the mercy of the health care system, willing to take on any debt to receive the gift of health. But sometimes, the price is too great causing many people to be buried in debt, which leads to bankruptcy, foreclosures, and housing problems.

Although the health care crisis may be out of control, there is still something that you can do to reduce the likelihood of ever needing the health care system, which is to increase your knowledge of food. It is imperative to your well-being to learn as much as possible to make informed decisions that may prove to be priceless over a lifetime.

Doctors

> *"The doctor of the future will give no medicine, but will*
> *interest his patients in the care of the human frame,*
> *and in the cause and prevention of disease."*
> — T. A. EDISON

After years of indulgence and self-neglect, many people expect doctors and pharmaceutical companies to improve their health. Medicine has made remarkable advancements, yet it is not infallible. Medical care is one of the top killers in the US. Health care-related errors kill more than 220,000 people per year and harm millions more.

Highly trained doctors misdiagnose adult patients 20 to 40% of the time and the percentage is even higher for children. Many doctors are overburdened and rush to see bushels of patients as an HMO requirement. Under these conditions many doctors cannot provide adequate guidance to help promote good health. Moreover, many doctors are ill-prepared to provide nutrition-related advice. Most medical schools devote less than 25 hours to the development of nutrition-related knowledge of doctors, leaving doctors poorly equipped to give good dietary advice. When nutrition-related instruction is given, most of the time it does not focus on prevention, but rather the biochemistry. Other times, nutrition is combined with other courses such as physiology and pharmacology. Nonetheless, nutrition does not receive the focused attention that it deserves. Not to mention that the food industry often supplies the nutrition-related educational material, which more than likely is a one-sided presentation of reality.

But doctors aren't the only ones who are not dedicated to nutrition education. In 2004, the National Institutes of Health dedicated only 3.6% of a 28 million dollar budget to nutrition, which is abysmal. Americans are in desperate need of good information that can help them make better health-related decisions; however, this should not be solely entrusted to tainted and limited sources.

There are close ties between the medical and pharmaceutical industries. Pharmaceutical companies start courting doctors with gifts and perks in medical schools to ensure devoted and profitable working relationships. And it doesn't stop there, once full-fledged doctors, pharmaceutical companies continue to shower doctors with gifts to encourage them to write prescriptions, even if it might not be in the best interest of the patients.

> *"It is easy to get a thousand prescriptions but*
> *hard to get one single remedy."*
> — CHINESE PROVERB

Doctors willingly write gads of prescriptions to individuals searching for solutions. Too much medication has a negative effect on the body. Overprescribed antibiotics lead to the development of antibiotic-resistant strains of bacteria, which are difficult to treat. Even if you are comfortable with taking pills to assuage health complications, improperly prescribed medications kill more than 100,000 people in the US every year. While a doctor can write you a prescription for any drug under the sun, a good diet is the only prescription that most people need.

There is an additional need for panic when dealing with drugs. Once drugs are approved by the FDA, doctors have carte blanche to write prescriptions. Unfortunately, at times doctors take the liberty to write the prescription off label, which means that the drug is being used for unintended purposes. This creates an additional source of problems. When drugs are prescribed for different uses not previously tested, there may be innumerable complications.

When not over-prescribing drugs, numerous doctors over-rely on surgeries to treat patients' health complications. A good diet may be a surgeon's last suggestion; the most likely solution may be you, a butcher knife, a butcher table, and lifetime regimen of pills. Cutting and prescriptions, it seems like it'd be easier to just make some modifications, but the easy way isn't for everyone. Leaving your life in the hands of a surgeon who gets paid to cut or a doctor who benefits from prescribing drugs is a questionable fate. Wouldn't you much rather take charge of your fate to ensure that you get the best possible result?

Many doctors' first reaction is to write a prescription or look for a surgical relief; however, nutrition may provide a more lasting effect, even a cure. Make every effort to avoid medical attention. Just being a patient in a hospital can worsen your condition if you fall prey to a nosocomial infection, which is an infection acquired in the hospital. Each year two million people acquire nosocomial infections and approximately 88,000 of them die. The hospital staff moves from sick person to sick person, which is the perfect opportunity to spread germs from patient to patient.

Pharmaceutical Companies and Drugs
*Consult your physician before changing any prescribed medicine.

> *"He that takes medicine and neglects diet,*
> *wastes the skill of the physician."*
> — CHINESE PROVERB

Some people would rather live it up today and pay the piper tomorrow. When the piper comes, many try to use the easy way out with drugs, and why not—there are so many wonder drugs available. At times it seems as though no matter what is ailing you, there is a pill for it. Pop it, and all is better. Failure to take proper care of yourself will mostly lead to a life dependent on expensive and interminable drugs. It is important to not blindly rely on the miracles and cures provided by the drug companies.

Granted, for a price drug companies provide wonderful services to millions dependent on their products for survival; however, drug companies have a vested interest in sickness. What better customer than the infirmed and forever dependent? Their miraculous products may be good, but they are no magic bullets. None of this is to say that the drug companies are a source of good or evil; however, their number one goal is profits, which is dependent on vast sickness.

Without properly managing your health, you are left to the mercy of the drug companies that prey on the illness of the sick. Americans currently spend over 30 billion dollars per year to bandage, not cure, self-inflicted damage from poor nutrition. Despite the relief that many drugs offer, they also contribute to further body deterioration.

"Cure the disease and kill the patient."
— Francis Bacon (1561–1626)

Drugs are powerful highly complex chemical concoctions. When desperate, drugs help those in need to hold on to life; however, there is always a trade-off when using drugs. While mending one portion of the body, drugs tend to have unwelcome side effects on other parts of the body. We've all heard the commercials announcing the endless side effects like: bloating, burning, coma, coughing, diarrhea, gas, heart attack, internal bleeding, itching, organ failure, respiratory complications, strokes, wheezing, vomiting, and death; but hey, the initial problem is gone. Although drugs may cause serious side effects, when faced with a death sentence, insane side effects don't seem so bad.

"Medicines are not meat to live by."
— German Proverb

Just because you don't need a prescription to take over-the-counter (OTC) medicines, does not mean that they are any safer than prescription drugs. Even the most common and benign drugs have incalculable, unintended side effects. OTCs affect the body's ability to naturally defend itself against maladies. Moreover, you may be doing more harm than good by masking the body's symptoms and thereby prolonging an aliment.

Prescriptions and OTC medications may limit the effectiveness of weight loss efforts. Everything that you put in your body is potentially the reason why you aren't losing weight. Before you pop your next pill, give it the twice over. Taking drugs generally produces an unwanted side effect like decreasing the rate food passes through the body, promoting constipation, reacting with other pills, perhaps leaving one or both ineffectual, and some drugs may reduce the body's ability to absorb nutrients. If you can, instead of popping pills, give your body what it really needs while leaving the pills bottle as mini maracas.

All drugs do not have the same effect. If you suspect your medication may interfere with your weight loss effort, then ask your doctor about other options.

Some medications that may impede weight loss include, but are not limited to:

+ Steroids
+ Antidepressants
+ Anticonvulsants
+ Birth control pills
+ Hormone replacement
+ Insulin and insulin stimulation

Medication may provide relief, but it alleviates the symptom, not the cause, which may do more harm than good. At times, it is best to allow the body the opportunity to heal itself because when you take drugs you are still left with the same problem, but now you have inundated your body with chemicals and it must fight the ailment and the chemicals. When infirmed, the body works diligently to eliminate illness and toxins through a series of actions like coughing, diarrhea, discharge, sweating, and vomiting. Many of the symptoms that the body displays are attempts to heal the body. But the body's healing process is too uncomfortable for most people and the quickest solution is sought. Have a cough? Take a cough suppressant; too bad if the body needs to dispel mucus, guess it's just going to sit there. Feeling too hot? Too bad if the body wants to kill pathogens by raising the temp a bit. Diarrhea? Take Pepto. Too bad the body wants to dispel infectious pathogens outside of the body. If you gotta go, let it go. Don't keep it in when it wants out.

Some medicines can effectively alleviate inflammation, pain, and symptoms for a short period of time; however, perpetual use can increase the likelihood of experiencing serious side effects. Toxic chemicals can kill tumors and surgery can remove them, but good nutrients have the power to reduce the likelihood of their existence. Diets have such a profound effect on health that prior disease may dissipate or even disappear with the nourishment of a good diet. That is getting to the root of the problem.

Pills

"A hypochondriac is one who has a pill for
everything except what ails him."
— MIGNON McLAUGHLIN,
THE SECOND NEUROTIC'S NOTEBOOK, 1966

Pills include a smorgasbord of contaminants known as excipients to help pills reach the right location and react in the body. The contents of pills include, but are not limited to:

+ **Antiadherents** reduce tablets from sticking to machinery molds.
+ **Binders** hold the pill's ingredients together. Common binders include: cellulose or modified cellulose such as microcrystalline cellulose, hydroxypropyl cellulose, lactose, starches, sugars, and sugar alcohols like maltitol, sorbitol, or xylitol.

- **Coatings** determine the point of disintegration, facilitate swallowing, and prevent deterioration. Common coatings include: cellulose, corn protein zein, shellac (plant fiber), or other polysaccharides.
- **Disintegrants** promote disintegration in specific parts of the body.
- **Fillers** enlarge a tablet or capsule with calcium carbonate, dibasic calcium phosphate, glucose, lactose, mannitol, plant cellulose, sorbitol, sucrose, vegetable fats and oils, and magnesium stearate to promote improved handling.
- **Flavors** enhance taste to ease ingestion.
- **Colors** enhance the appearance and promote identification of the medication.
- **Glidants** facilitate ingestion by reducing friction and cohesion. Glidants include colloidal silicon dioxide and talc.
- **Lubricants** prevent ingredients from clumping and sticking to the pill cutter a.k.a. tablet puncher or capsule filling machine.
- **Preservatives** increase shelf life and reduce rancidness. Common preservatives include: citric acid, cysteine, methionine, retinyl palmitate, selenium, sodium citrate, vitamin A, vitamin C, vitamin E, and methyl- and propyl paraben.
- **Sorbents** protect against moisture.
- **Sweeteners** mask and improve the taste and smell.

All of these can be in a single pill. Geez! After ingesting all of this, you might need a diet.

Even the most common and regularly used pills may cause side effects.

- Antibiotics—diarrhea, nausea, vomiting, and fungal infections of the mouth, digestive tract, and vagina from destroying the resident 'good' bacteria in the body while killing the 'bad' infection.

+ Antihistamines—dizziness, nervousness, restlessness, and upset stomach. Rare side effects include: blurred vision, difficulty urinating, dry mouth, dry nose, and irritability.
+ Antiviral—agitation, anxiety, delirium, difficulty concentrating, genetic mutation, hallucinations, light-headedness, nausea, nervousness, and seizures.
+ Aspirin—heartburn, nausea, and upset stomach.
+ Aspirin with codeine—constipation, diarrhea, dizziness, drowsiness, headache, indigestion, light-headedness, mild stomach pain, nausea, and vomiting.
+ Birth control pills—bleeding, blood clots, breast tenderness, cancer, headache, increased blood pressure, irregular bleeding, mood swings, nausea, stroke, and weight gain.
+ NSAIDs — constipation, decreased appetite, diarrhea, dizziness, drowsiness, headache, nausea, rash, and vomiting. NSAIDs may also cause fluid retention and lead to edema. The most serious side effects are kidney and liver failure, prolonged bleeding after an injury or surgery, and ulcers.
+ Steroids—delusions, extreme irritability, fluid retention, high blood pressure, impaired judgment, jaundice, liver tumors, and paranoid jealousy.
  ◇ Men: baldness, development of breasts, infertility, reduced sperm count, and smaller testicles.
  ◇ Women: changes in the menstrual cycle, deepened voice, and growth of facial hair.
  ◇ Adolescents: stunted growth.

Pharmaceutical companies focus on the drugs that will generate at least $500 million in sales per year and prominence by developing drugs for large spread long-term ailments to ensure consumers remain dependent year after year. With that in mind, pharmaceutical companies focus on allergies, Alzheimer's, anxiety, arthritis, depression, diabetes, high cholesterol, obesity, and osteoporosis; almost all of which research has found to be improved by a good diet. But why ruin a good business with a few simple modifications?

Although drug companies provide miracle drugs to those in desperate need of assistance, they are far from being a goody two shoes. They are in it to win it, and to do it they spend over three billion dollars in multi-platform advertising designed to motivate the public to request doctors to write prescriptions that lead to 200 billion dollars in sales. Only the US and New Zealand have direct-to-consumer advertising due to the fact that it causes a series of problems like manipulating people into thinking they have a variety of health problems from the incomplete information provided by advertising. Although, it may be educational to provide the public with information, it often causes more harm than good. Nonetheless, the commercials are somewhat effective because over 30% of 1,222 people surveyed replied that they asked their doctor about drugs seen in recent advertising, over 25% asked for a prescription, of which over 70% were awarded prescriptions. Advertising can be very manipulative. Many consumers are swayed by advertising. Consumers must be aware of the influence leveraged from third-party endorsements.

It seems as though drug companies will do just about anything to keep the profits in the billions, like create a new drug (Clarinex), which is basically the same as their last drug (Claritin) because their patent is running out and they won't be able to collect exorbitant profits. Or perhaps pay off generic drug makers to ensure they don't manufacture a drug whose patent has run out, which will reduce the patent holder's profits. Or maybe sue a generic drug maker to extend the patent holder's right to sale the patented expensive version of the drug; with few or no generic drug makers, prescription drugs can remain expensive and generate mega profits.

Drug companies spend an estimated 850 million to 1.2 billion dollars and 12 years of experimentation and trials to prepare a drug for public use. Such a grand investment may encourage ruthlessness and frenzied motivation to get the drug on the market through any means necessary, at least to recoup of few funds if the drug is taken off the market by the FDA (Food and Drug Administration).

While in the drug development stage, drug companies do testing; however, drugs are tested on a limited amount of people, for a limited amount of time, and not all side effects are apparent during the trial. More complete information concerning the way a drug may affect individuals is learned after the drug is FDA approved and available for everyone through a doctor's prescription for months—even years.

Unfortunately some people may be stricken with multiple conditions like high blood pressure and diabetes. During the clinical trials, it is time and cost-prohibitive to review the reactions among multiple drugs and health complications. Unfortunately, when people take several prescriptions for multiple ailments, basically all hell could break loose inside the body.

Pharmaceuticals offer relief from symptoms, but wouldn't it be better if you could take steps to avoid them altogether? At times drug companies may seem like miracle makers, but they're profit-oriented businesses. Drug companies don't invest millions of dollars to find natural cures; they create complex patentable chemical solutions that may have unidentified negative side effects. Yes, it is nice to have a medical professional to assist you; however, with so many agendas and uncertainties revolving around health care it is imperative to arm yourself with information and be an advocate for yourself.

Food and Drug Administration (FDA)

"It would be nice if the Food and Drug Administration
stopped issuing warnings about toxic substances and just
gave me the names of one or two things still safe to eat."
— ROBERT FUOSS
EXEC. ED. 'SATURDAY EVENING POST', 1956–61

After pharmaceutical companies have invested years and millions of dollars into a drug in hopes of developing the next super drug, there is just one thing between them and the public's billions—the FDA. The Food and Drug Administration (FDA) is an arm of the government that works to protect the public's health by determining the safeness of biologics, cosmetics, foods, human and veterinary drugs, medical devices, and radiation products. The public is very dependent on the FDA's protection. Generally, the public believes drugs and foods are safe because they have been approved by the FDA. Many people blindly trust that the FDA takes all of the necessary precautions to ensure their well-being, but this does not always happen.

Bextra, Bromfeac, Celebrex, Crestor, Fen-Phen, Meridia, Mibefradil, Serevan, Terfenadine, Troglitazane, and Vioxx are a few among the countless drugs that received the FDA's seal of approval that later released a litany of horror on the unsuspecting public. People who blindly relied on the strict scrutiny of the FDA suffered injury and even death. Even more appalling are the many warning signs that were unfortunately ignored during and after the drug approval process. It appears as though, after a drug has been approved, the FDA only recalls drugs after catastrophic loss occurs.

To be approved, new drugs only have to be more effective than sugar pills. Never mind that the drug may cause a slew of problems or a better product may already exist on the market; that is not the FDA's concern. Each year, drugs approved by the FDA kill more than 100,000 people, but the CDC does not permit this category of death. Another 1.5 million escape the clutches of death, but require hospitalization.

Reviewers at the FDA are expected to review thousands of pages of drug documentation in limited amounts of time. Many employees at the FDA are not comfortable voicing concerns over the safety of drugs submitted by the big pharmaceutical companies and some who have voiced concerns received punishments.

In the late 1980s, there were several felony convictions of FDA drug reviewers who had been paid by drug companies to approve their drugs. Researchers working on pharmaceuticals and artificial sweeteners have acknowledged doing the following:

+ Falsifying data
+ Concealing negative data
+ Insufficient record keeping
+ Concealing conflicts of interest
+ Utilizing an inferior research design
+ Implementing the wrong research design

On the other hand, while many people are grateful for the FDA's zealous, in-depth inspection, gravely ill individuals knocking on death's door would like a chance at life and that means trying new drugs that may offer hope. Although pharmaceutical companies allow some individuals to participate in their drug trials, everyone does not receive this opportunity, so they have to wait until the drug hits the market, which may be too late.

As part of the approval process, pharmaceutical companies pay the FDA to review their drug; however, it appears as though some pharmaceutical companies interpret this collaboration as a guaranteed paid approval.

The FDA is under considerable pressure from multiple fronts. Pharmaceutical companies spend in the ballpark of 150 million dollars to influence legislation, five million dollars of which is directed at the FDA. As if the pressures from the pharmaceutical companies were not enough, it is estimated that Congress sends more than 200 inquiries to the FDA per year about the progress of certain drugs, which may undoubtedly be an effort to rush the process. Despite the intentions of the FDA, its power is limited and succumbing to formidable political pressures may be inevitable.

Research

> *Research is what I'm doing when I don't know what I'm doing.*
> — WERNHER VON BRAUN

Each industry (Big Pharma, Big Sugar, Big Tobacco, etc.) employs their own team of lobbyists, scientists, and statisticians to attest to the value of their products. These giants encourage their team to demonstrate the safeness and worthiness of their product, which is not hard. Scientists and statisticians can make any data look good. The average American does not have the expertise or even access to the data to examine the validity of most research studies.

Although researchers should operate under strict ethics to ensure accurate and unbiased results for the safety of the public, this does not always happen. Research reports carry significant value and improve products' marketability. To the public, research studies serve as an unbiased source of information that can be trusted.

Vitamins

> *"You can't buy health out of a bottle."*
> — UNKNOWN

Food contains macronutrients and micronutrients to build, maintain, and repair the cellular components of the body. Macronutrients (macro—big) include carbohydrates, fats, protein, and water; the body requires more than one gram of these nutrients per day. While micronutrients (micro—small) provide vitamins and minerals, the body requires less than one gram of these nutrients per day.

Vitamins are carbon-containing compounds required by the body in minuscule amounts to carry out metabolic functions. That is why a well-balanced diet is so important. As the body of knowledge regarding diseases grows, many ailments appear to be diseases of deficiency of essential nutrients. Deficiencies are not common when a variety of foods are consumed. Therefore, it is important not to rely on any one source of food. Essential nutrients cannot be manufactured by the body; they must be obtained from food or supplements. Fruits and vegetables are a storehouse of vitamins, minerals, and antioxidants that may be able to prevent illness and the degeneration of the body. Without the necessary nutrients, the body may use an inappropriate replacement or may not carry out necessary functions.

The vitamins that researchers have identified as pivotal to good health have been extracted from the cumbersome, meddlesome, bothersome fruits and vegetables and refined to make a vitamin supplement. Vitamins known to be essential to health include:

Vitamin A	Vitamin K	Vitamin B_2	Folate
Vitamin D	Vitamin C	Vitamin B_6	Niacin
Vitamin E	Vitamin B_1	Vitamin B_{12}	Folate
Biotin		Pantothenic acid	

Vitamins that dissolve in water are known as water-soluble. Water-soluble vitamins are not stored in the body. The body absorbs the water-soluble vitamins needed and the rest are excreted in urine. Water-soluble vitamins include vitamins B and C. On the other hand, fat-soluble vitamins dissolve in fat and are stored in the body. Fat-soluble vitamins include vitamins A, D, E, and K.

Vitamin supplements, as well as medications, can be very beneficial under certain conditions. Supplements serve as insurance to ensure essential vitamins and minerals are provided daily, which is wonderful for people who aren't able to get adequate nutrition to help maintain their health like: breastfeeders, crazy restrictive dieters, infirmed, menopausers, pregnant women, and smokers. Supplements provide a great service; however, they are not panaceas and will not ensure good health.

Millions of dollars are spent each year by consumers who want the benefits of vitamins. How many pills are you willing to swallow to lose weight and gain health? There are many reasons why people take vitamin supplements like they provide essential nutrients, some people believe they offer incalculable curing abilities, others try to alleviate the negative effects of a bad diet by taking vitamin supplements, but mostly everyone loves the easy fix. Planning and eating a diet filled with nutritious food is too cumbersome for some people. Why eat well? Just pop one pill and you're free to do and eat anything you want while being healthy. Not quite. The dangers of unhealthy diets cannot be reversed by popping pills.

Some people are addicted to the promise of vitality that vitamin supplements provide and they swallow them by the truckloads. Many people have heard about the wonderful effects that antioxidants have on the body and have decided to maximize the benefits by consuming more antioxidant supplements. Antioxidants like vitamin C and E are known to neutralize free radicals that wreak havoc inside of the body. One celebrity went on a national talk show proclaiming she takes 20+ vitamin supplements a day to promote her health and vitality. The stellar results of natural foods are not always replicated by synthetic means in the body. Some researchers have found that there are not any health benefits from taking synthetic antioxidants, while others have even found taking supplements can actually have negative effects such as cardiovascular complications.

Vitamin supplements promise nutrients in a nice little package, but they offer less good than you may have expected. Vitamin supplements aren't very tasty and contain ingredients like coatings, binding agents, preservatives, shells, and starches; all of which are foreign elements that further complicate digestion, bodily functions, and metabolism. At times, the body is not able to successfully eliminate all substances and stores them, even if they are harmful. Over time, the storage of chemicals and toxins has a negative effect on the body. Therefore, careful consideration should be given to everything ingested.

Vitamin supplements are a great gamble. What you see is not always what you get. The quality and potency of vitamin supplements can vary widely between brands and manufacturers. Vitamin supplements do not sustain the scrutiny of prescription drugs and may be made of inferior synthetic ingredients, rather than pure substances. Multiple brands of vitamins have tested positive for pesticides and toxins like cancer-causing polychlorinated biphenyls (PCBs).

The journey of nutrients to form a vitamin supplement is a long and arduous process that may involve chemicals, grinding, heating, and processing, thereby significantly reducing the nutrients. Vitamins are very delicate and are negatively affected by virtually everything like coatings, heat, light, moisture, and oxidation, which causes them to lose potency from the moment they are made until they are worthless. In fact, by the time some vitamins are sold they may have lost up to 50% of their potency. To retain the potency of the vitamin supplement at home it is important to store them in a cool dry place.

There are several important factors to consider when purchasing vitamins. Look for the GMP logo (Good Manufacturing Processing), which ensures the quality of vitamin supplements through inspections and testing the ingredients. Review the expiration date to ensure the supplement has not expired.

Carefully review the label to help determine the quality of the vitamins. For instance, the label may say natural vitamins, yet contain a significant amount of synthetic vitamins, which are cheaper to manufacture and easily destroyed by stomach acids. Although powdered and liquid concentrations of vitamins are recommended; whole foods have more nutrients.

Consume the right recommended dietary allowance (RDA) of vitamin supplements. Although supplements may provide wonderful nutrients, it is possible to take too many supplements. More is not always best; in fact, ingesting too many supplements can be detrimental to your health. Carefully monitor taking new supplements. Some supplements may have a negative effect so slight that it may be too late when noticed.

All vitamin supplements must be carefully balanced. Vitamins are not consistently absorbed once ingested. Taken incorrectly, vitamins can be completely useless and excreted from the body without being absorbed. Follow the instructions and recommendations to ensure nutrients within the supplements are absorbed. Natural sources have better bioavailability, which is the ease of which the vitamin is absorbed into the body.

Mega doses are pretty unlikely on a regular diet; however, taking multivitamins supplements increases the likelihood of a mega dose. Also, the possibility of a vitamin overdose is increased if you eat or drink vitamin enriched cereal, fortified milk, or nutrient rich food. Research studies have shown that vitamins taken in high dosages actually promote health complications, instead of reducing them. Studies show that previously safe recommended amounts of vitamins have been linked to overdoses causing weakened bones and hip fractures.

There are studies that show that excessive supplements like vitamins A, B_6 and E may be harmful to good health. Increased consumption of vitamin A may cause birth defects and symptoms associated with brain tumors. Increased consumption of B_6 may cause temporary nerve damage; however, there aren't any studies that report too many fruits or vegetables are bad for health.

Anything ingested has the ability to interact with everything in the body. All drugs have the ability to interfere with the effectiveness of other pills. Drugs and foods have the ability to increase or decrease the effectiveness of vitamin supplements, and vice versa. Too much of a vitamin may inhibit the absorption of other minerals and vitamins; too little may inhibit the absorption of another vitamin and may promote deficiencies.

You could get nutrients in the form of pills, but then you'd miss out on all of the other vitamins and minerals that come in whole foods. Despite all of the good intentions of supplements, the complex nature of whole unrefined fruits and vegetables cannot be precisely replicated by artificial means. Natural unprocessed foods pack a wealth of good inside of them; some of the good has not even been identified yet. Every day it seems as though additional benefits of natural unprocessed food are identified as the miracle source to improve health and reduce the risk of disease. Vitamin supplements are infinitely inferior to natural sources of foods. If you really want to impact your health and give your body a super duper treat that will help it function in optimal condition—eliminate the middle man; get your vitamins right from the source in the form of fruits and vegetables. A well-balanced diet is the best way to get all of your vitamins and nutrients.

Minerals

Unlike vitamins, which are organic, minerals are inorganic atoms that are naturally found in rocks and metal ores. Minerals found in plants and animals were obtained from mineral-rich soil. Like vitamins, minerals can interfere with the effectiveness of drugs. Minerals provide important support to bodily functions. Adequate levels of magnesium are required to provide sufficient energy. Magnesium absorption is reduced by excess insulin, which is consistently produced with high sugar consumption. Magnesium is found fruits and grains. Chromium helps insulin work effectively. Studies have shown that adequate chromium intake enhances weight loss efforts. Major essential minerals are:

Calcium	Magnesium	Potassium	Sulfur
Chloride	Phosphorus	Sodium	

Herbal Supplements

Herbal supplements are quite popular, which may be attributed to the numerous feigned claims of improved health and vitality. Many people falsely assume herbal supplements are safe because they are natural; however, there is good cause to be wary about herbal supplements, especially if you are taking any additional drugs including OTCs. Herbal supplements may cause serious complications when taken with any other drug. There have been many serious side effects from taking herbal supplements including, but not limited to: cancer, rashes, strokes, and liver and kidney damage. But there is a bright side; once a significant amount of people get sick or die from consuming a herbal supplement, the FDA intervenes and bans the sale of the product. Hey, better late than never or you can just say no to herbal concoctions. There is no substitute for a good diet.

Conclusion

Although you might look to the FDA or another alternative source of assistance to look out for your health interest, you must be the primary decision maker for your health. Profit-oriented businesses have alternative motives for their actions and recommendations that may not be in your best interest. Unfortunately you cannot get good health from a pill, from a doctor, pharmacy, or by magical means; you have to earn it. If illness sets in, you may be at the mercy of doctors, drug companies, and pills for the rest of your life.

While taking supplements can provide your body with essential nutrients to prevent illness, it is important to remember that supplements are only able to provide a limited supply of nutrients that may cause negative side effects within the body. The best sources of vitamins and minerals are whole unrefined plant products. Plant products provide the body with the nutrients needed while avoiding overdoses and side effects that may occur when taking vitamin supplements.

There are steps that you can immediately take to reduce the likelihood of being dependent on the less than perfect alternatives. Now we going to look at multiple diets and explore why they are a bad idea and may not be a permanent solution for anyone. Don't fret; once you know why they didn't work, you will also learn what will work. Let's go!

Why Diets Don't Work 4

"A diet is the penalty we pay for exceeding the feed limit."
— UNKNOWN

EXCESS WEIGHT IS SO imprisoning that many people take drastic measures to get rid of it. Most of us have tried more diets than we care to admit, in an attempt to lose the extra pounds that keep us from feeling and looking our best. There are tons of weight loss diets, but not all of them are safe, nor will they provide lasting, maintainable, healthy results. The meat diet, the no meat diet, the lemon diet, the quick diet, the super quick quick diet. Everyone wants immediate results, and that may be the reason for the emergence of so many creative diet approaches. Although creative, almost all of them have significant flaws.

Many people apply effort, yet never realize the fruits of their labor, which can be very discouraging. Others experience the sad cycle of yo-yo dieting; losing some weight, but only to gain it back with additional pounds; this cycle is not good for your body or health. Many diets can help dieters be successful temporarily, but who wants the taste of success for seconds? A more permanent solution is needed.

We are a nation that loves easy solutions, but they are not always permanent, satisfying, maintainable, or healthy. Searching for a weight loss solution, many people try one fad diet after another. It is very tempting to be lured in by the promise of big weight loss guaranteed by fad diets; however, there is always a catch. If it looks too good to be true, it probably is. Most fad diets aren't healthy and may cause a series of issues including, but not limited to: bloating, constipation, depression, fatigue, hair loss, hunger, insomnia, intense cravings, nervousness, skin problems, and weak nails.

Most fad diets don't promote significant and lasting weight loss because they are missing basic elements to be successful. Your diet has to do everything. It has to be livable day in and day out; if it is not, you may abandon it like a sinking ship. Too many diets shortsightedly focus on weight loss. It is not enough that your diet helps you lose weight, but it also must be healthy, easily maintainable, satisfying, and flexible to mesh well with your life. If any one of these vital components is missing, your diet may end in disaster. You many initially lose weight, but more than likely the weight is not gone for good, but rather vacationing and waiting to come back with a couple of other pounds.

You can't stop eating just because you're on a diet; well, you can, but it doesn't feel good and it probably won't work. There is only so long your stomach or brain is going to remain hungry before your diet plan is abandoned. The body has plans of its own called survival, which requires food. Eating also keeps your metabolism going. When sustenance is low, there is a greater likelihood that your metabolism will slow. You can't stay on a diet if you're hungry, and you shouldn't expect yourself to.

Being overweight is not just about how much you eat, it is also about what you eat. How many times have you said to yourself "I really haven't eaten that much," but you still don't lose weight? All too often people quickly assess the cause of being overweight is simply attributed to eating too much and lack of exercise. If only it were that easy.

Ninety-nine percent of diets don't help you live in the real world—they try to make you participate in some alternate universe where your meals are turned upside down and inside out for weight loss. And for good reason, they make money off of your dependence. They want you to come back time and time again after you lose your way.

There are so many crazy diets available concocted of a little of this and little of that, which generally makes no sense or does more harm than good—even if you could lose weight by following them, most of them are devoid of the nutrients needed to promote health. There will always be a fad diet that guarantees fast weight loss. Most diets operate basically the same way with a slight twist or a pinch of insanity here and there. Let's explore some of the flaws of popular diets and why they will not work for long or at all.

Commando Diets

| Flexible | ★ | Healthy | ★ | Maintainable | ★ | Satisfying | ★ |

Commando diets promise big rewards if you follow an insanely strict diet. Generally, commando diets focus on losing mega amounts fast. The diet operates under the guise if a rigorous and strict diet is followed then weight loss is bound to occur. To this end, commando diets require strict dieting, which may not provide enough nutrients to maintain a healthy body. Flexibility is MIA with commando diets. As you already know, life happens and you have to adjust and move on to the next challenge. Adhering to a strict and outrageous diet is not feasible for the average person.

Die-hard dieters believe it has to be all or nothing. But this is not true. We all know someone who has lived well, despite a bad habit here and there. And of course when we remind naysayers of this truth, they say, "that is the exception, not the rule." Well pooh-pooh on them, we all can still learn something from the exception.

Moderation is key; a life devoid of pleasure doesn't seem like much fun, but adding goodness to your diet can balance out the naughty here and there. Commando diets aren't for anyone who enjoys eating a morsel of food. Commando diets will continually leave you hungry and dissatisfied and impatiently waiting for the end of your diet. Commando diets are not easily maintainable because you are so hungry, temptation will be everywhere; there is nowhere that you can hide where food will not be calling your name. You have to be satisfied in order to stick with your weight loss plan.

Counting Calories

| Flexible | ★★★ | Healthy | ★★ | Maintainable | ★★ | Satisfying | ★★★ |

Counting calories scrutinizes calorie consumption to promote weight loss. Basically there are 3,500 calories per pound, which can easily be eaten in one day; but not easily taken off in one day. So how do these pounds add up? Fat has nine calories per gram, while protein and carbohydrates have four calories per gram. Therefore, by eating vegetables and fruits you eliminate hunger and add fiber to your diet while consuming fewer calories. A hundred grams of fatty food will give you 900 calories, while eating the same amount of protein or carbohydrate will give you 400 calories. By choosing healthier options, you actually get to eat more food. Over a year, that can make a big difference in the waistline.

Food	Calories per gram
Protein	4
Carbohydrates	4
Oil	9
Fat	9
Alcohol	7

For example, if a woman utilizes 1,500 calories per day, consumes 1,200 calories per day diet, theoretically, she is eating 300 fewer calories than her body requires. If the woman sticks to the diet, by the end of the week she has lost a whopping two-thirds of a pound. This rate sounds like a slow arduous process, but not really; that is exactly how the weight crept on. A half pound one week, one-third of a pound the next. No one gains 20 pounds overnight, thankfully.

Calorie counting diets can be flexible; however, the challenge is tracking and calculating the caloric content of every morsel of food that enters your mouth throughout the day. Everything counts, from the juice at breakfast, the samples at the grocery store, and the chips you nibbled on.

While knowing the caloric background of food is beneficial, calorie counting can be very tricky; calorie contents may be difficult to determine, especially when eating out and adding sides and condiments. Many restaurants do not readily provide caloric information on their menu items. In addition, there may be errors in the assessment of calories. For instance, a dish may be advertised at 1,000 calories per serving. However, portion sizes may vary, concealing extra calories. The weekend chef may give out 50% more food. Is that a good or bad thing? More food, but more calories. Without a calorimeter it may be impossible to know the amount of calories consumed, and is thereby misleading. Dieters need a more practical way to lose weight.

You can lose weight eating anything if you limit the amount of calories you consume. If your body requires 1,300 calories per day, and you only eat 650 calories of cheesecake—you're losing more than a pound per week, but you're not improving your health. While counting calories may address the caloric content of food, it does not address the nutritional content. Without the proper nutrients, your body may not run optimally or lose weight. Any diet can lead to weight loss, but it is important that it does not damage your health in the process.

Daily calorie consumption recommendations from the USDA are as follows:

+ Seniors—1,600 calories per day
+ Children—1,600 calories per day
+ Inactive women—1,600 calories per day
+ Inactive men—2,200 calories per day
+ Moderately active women—2,200 calories per day
+ Teenage girls—2,200 calories per day
+ Teenage boys—2,800 calories per day
+ Active men—2,800 calories per day
+ Active women—2,800 calories per day
+ Pregnant and lactating women—2,200 to 2,800 calories per day

According to National Institutes of Health, to lose weight women should consume less than 1,200 calories, and men should consume less than 1,600 calories. While specific daily calorie recommendations may be accurate for some people, the recommendations do not take into account build, height, weight, or all of the variables that can have a significant effect on calorie usage. Metabolisms vary from person to person each day. Everyone is different; the amount of calories a body requires each day to do basic activities varies depending on a multitude of factors.

Precise measurement of all meals is not feasible or necessary; however, food consumption should fall into the following range:

+ Protein—2 to 10%
+ Saturated fats—10% or less
+ Mono and polyunsaturated fat—15 to 20%
+ Carbohydrates (including fiber) — 60 to 70% of calories

Depending on how many calories you are allotting yourself, this can look different. Calorie requirements differ depending on age, gender, hormones, level of activity, and metabolism.

Lower-calorie diets

	1,000	1,250	1,500
Saturated fats	100	1250	150
Mono & polyunsaturated fats	150–200	200–260	225–300
Carbohydrates (+ fiber)	600–700	750–875	900–1,050
Protein	20–100	25–125	30–150

Higher-calorie diets

	1,750	2,000	2,250
Saturated fats	175	200	225
Mono & Polyunsaturated fats	263–350	300–400	338–450
Carbohydrates (+ fiber)	1,050–1,225	1,200–1,400	1,350–1,575
Protein	35–175	40–200	45–225

There are basically three main types of food groups known as carbohydrates, fats, and proteins. These three groups can be further dichotomized into healthy and unhealthy groups, whereas if you only ate food out of the unhealthy groups, you may feel satisfied, but weight loss may not happen and you may experience an increased risk of illness.

While more in-depth information will be provided ahead, basically all fat is not completely bad. Saturated fat is unhealthy while unsaturated fat is better. Straight from the ground fruits and vegetables are infinitely healthier than refined and processed carbohydrates, yet both are carbohydrates. While meat is not the only source of protein, it is a complete source. Plant products provide protein and so many more beneficial nutrients.

Dieting should not be as hard as algebra with computations of calories; it should be painless and effortless to maintain. The best diet is flexible and promotes good health. Don't worry about counting calories. If you eat the right food, generally you can eat as much as you like while losing weight and avoiding the torturous pain of an empty stomach.

Diet Pills

Flexible	★	Healthy	★	Maintainable	★	Satisfying	★

There are a series of weight loss drugs and medications that are available to suppress appetite, reduce fat absorption, increase metabolism, and induce bowel movements; however, the results are less than stellar for the risks involved. Not to mention, none of the weight loss drugs enhance weight loss after they are discontinued. Permanent and significant weight loss generally will not occur from popping pills. Achieving weight loss may be especially difficult without a good diet and exercise. Some diet pills require a particular diet while other diet pills allow dieters to feast on anything. Diet pills may offer a fair amount of flexibility for food selections; however, eating healthier food selections may enhance your results.

OTC weight loss pills come with a barrel of side effects like diarrhea, elevated blood pressure, elevated heart rate, nervousness, tremors, and even heart failure. OTC weight loss pills may result in serious health complications including, but not limited to: anxiety, cardiac complications, depression, headaches, high blood pressure, psychosis, and mental and physical addiction.

In addition to all of the hazards that come with diet pills, they have additional dangers. Diet pills have been in play since the 1950s. Back then patients were prescribed amphetamines, which is basically speed. Some of the other drugs promising better bods were Fenfluramine (Pondimin), dexfenfluramine (Redux), a phentermine, and later a combination of phentermine and Fenfluramine. All of these drugs had the approval of the FDA, but were later removed from the market after reports of serious health complications. The FDA approves weight loss medications, only to find out months, even years later that they are unsafe and may have devastating consequences. Ephedra supplements caused hundreds of negative reactions including dizziness, heart attacks, nausea, seizures, and strokes, which later caused a warning to be issued about the drug.

Diet drugs typically recommend a sensible diet with exercise while providing negligible enhancements of maybe 5 to 7% additional weight loss, which may be achieved through good ole diet and exercise alone. So why are diet pills so popular? Drug companies know that many people are desperate to lose weight and are willing to capitalize on that fact.

Diet pills may help to suppress the urge to eat, which may help dieters get control over their appetite to promote weight loss, but they will likely have a negative effect on the body. Even when appetite suppression is successful, drastically reducing calories may slow down the metabolism and limit weight loss.

Right in line with the magical cure we find fat blockers. Swallow a fat blocker pill and you'll be able to eat all of the fat that you want without gaining weight. Not! Although fat blockers promote weight loss for a while, they have not been effective for significant periods of time. Not to mention, they have some pretty nasty side effects like diarrhea, oily stools, and unexpected fecal discharge. Yikes! Break out the diapers. To reduce the negative side effects, dieters are encouraged to eat a low-fat diet or face a fecal discharge in public. Jinkees! Fat blockers also inhibit the body's ability to absorb fat-soluble vitamins like A, D, E, and K. There are also carb blockers that prevent the absorption of carbohydrates. Sounds great, but these little wonders come with the price of unexpected emissions like gas and more.

At best, diet pills may be used to kick-start weight loss; however, everything ingested has the potential to promote internal damage as well as decrease metabolism. Diet pills are basically a risky gamble and unless serious changes are made after weight loss is attained, the results may not be permanent.

Glycemic Index

Flexible	★★	Healthy	★★	Maintainable	★★	Satisfying	★★

The glycemic index diet attempts to preemptively manage sugar levels by utilizing an index to identify how carbohydrates may impact the body's sugar or glucose levels. Carbohydrates are easily broken down into sugar, which significantly affects blood sugar levels. The way that the body processes sugar determines if sugar is used or stored. If the body is able to properly manage sugar, then there will not be high levels of sugar in the blood, alleviating the need to store excess as fat. A major part of managing blood sugar is selecting food that will not significantly raise it. The pancreas produces insulin to reduce the amount of sugar circulating in the blood and ushers sugar to the cells where it is needed. Bodies that are not able to properly reduce blood sugar levels develop diabetes and other complications.

High glycemic index foods generally include refined and simple carbs. Refined and simple carbs are easily digested causing blood sugar to rise rapidly. Carbs that increase blood sugar rapidly, also decrease it rapidly, creating an urge to eat sooner, rather than later. On the other hand, low glycemic index foods like complex carbs, including starches and legumes take longer to digest, which releases glucose gradually and has a more level effect on blood sugar. The gradual release of glucose is thought to help dieters and diabetics stay satisfied longer, while helping to regulating blood sugar.

When following the glycemic index diet it is important to determine the glycemic load in an attempt to predict how carbs will affect blood sugar. To calculate the glycemic load, multiply the grams of available carbs in a serving and the index value, then divide by 100. This might be a little more investigating and calculating than you'd like to do each time you eat.

Glycemic Load	
Low	≤ 10
Medium	11–19
High	20+

The glycemic diet recommends meals based on a lower glycemic load than the body requires to hopefully result in weight loss. To lose weight, glycemic index experts recommend a glycemic load or 60–75 per day. A typical daily diet may include three meals with a glycemic load of 15, and two snacks with a glycemic load of 10; however, this general diet recommendation may need adjustment to account for different metabolic rates and how each body reacts to carbohydrates. If weight loss does not occur; additional decreases in glycemic load are generally recommended. You can go lower, but less than 40 grams per day is not recommended. Carbohydrates are an important part of the diet, and further carbohydrate restrictions may do more harm than good.

Although glycemic index fans like the scientific-ness of the glycemic index diet, it is a far cry from a complete and accurate science. There are many uncertainties and unknown variables that significantly impede the reliability of the diet, which makes it difficult for some dieters to achieve success.

The glycemic index provides a variety of unrefined and unprocessed plant products, which can be healthy and satisfying; however, the index is quite limited and does not take all foods like meats and oils into consideration. Meats and oils are a huge part of the American diet, but are basically ignored. Discounting the impact of meats and fats on the diet is a mistake because they pack significant calories. Adequate dietary precautions must be taken, even though they don't have a significant impact on blood sugar. If any foods not listed on the index are eaten, you've basically abandoned the diet and you are on your own. Although carbs play an important role in the diet equation, they are definitely not the whole picture.

There is some flexibility in the glycemic index diet. The index provide a list of foods along with their values for you to select from; however, the problems start when you deviate slightly from a single food listed on the index because combining and mixing foods may have untold effects on blood sugar from person to person.

Low Glycemic Index	Medium Glycemic Index	High Glycemic Index
≤ 55	56–69	≥ 70
Complex carbs, fiber, and grains	White sugar	Refined carbs and white flour

Research studies have found carbohydrates have different effects on everyone's blood sugar. For example, eating a banana may raise one person's blood sugar by 10, another person's by 15, and another person's by 5. The glycemic index takes an average of how carbohydrates affect the blood sugar of multiple individuals. In this case the average would be 10 and a value of 10 would be placed on the glycemic index—only an example. If it so happens that 10 is really the amount that a banana raises your blood sugar, lucky you; however, if it's not, your calculations for the day may be off. Oops!

On the glycemic index, high fructose corn syrup rates low, anywhere from a 10 to 32. While many nutrient-rich fruits like cantaloupe, carrots, papaya, and watermelon have earned a medium to high rating, this essentially equates those foods as junk food, despite their rich nutritional value. The erratic index misnomers many foods, and has the potential to cause harm to anyone who may trustingly follow the recommendation of the glycemic index.

Although there have been improvements in understanding how foods affect glucose levels in the body, it is a very complex calculation that is still not perfectly understood. Certain foods like fats and cinnamon unexplainably lower blood sugar. In addition, there aren't any accurate results of alcohol's effect on blood sugar because the results can be different before, during, and after consuming alcohol from person to person. Combining carbohydrates with fats and protein creates an even greater problem with the glycemic diet. Multiple foods change the effect on the body's blood sugar. So at best, it is a guesstimate. Despite changes, revisions, and updates to the glycemic index, the total effect of carbohydrates on the body is not understood.

It would be fantastic to have a magic formula to help determine what should be on the menu, but this is not it. With so many unknown and unexplainable variables and calculations, it may be better to leave this diet to the omniscient. If healthy food selections are chosen, there is basically no need for the glycemic index.

Meat Diet

Flexible	★	Healthy	★	Maintainable	★★★	Satisfying	★★★

Diets generally leave most people unsatisfied and craving the next morsel of food, but not the meat diet. The meat diet can satisfy hunger like no other diet, but satisfaction isn't everything.

Unlike specialty diets with hard to find delicacies, surviving on the meat diet is fairly easy in the US culture where there are many different forms of meat to choose at grocery stores, restaurants, or fast food establishments.

Flexibility is limited with meat diet. The diet basically consists of meat and little else because once carbohydrates are eaten, the body reverts back to processing them. Although meat satisfies hunger well, the body requires and may even crave a wider variety of nutrients to satisfy its nutritional needs.

Many dietary researchers recommend limiting animal products to 10% of the daily caloric intake. Moreover, they claim that health can be improved if the consumption of animal products is reduced to one or two servings per week.

You might lose weight adhering to a meat diet, but it will cost you your health. Some of the weight that is lost on a meat diet can be attributed to water weight, because ketosis resembles a diuretic. Under regular conditions, the body obtains its fuel from carbohydrates, which are easily broken down into glucose. But a diet of all meat alters the body's preferred modus operatus. So the body goes into ketosis, an adaptive survival mode to metabolize fat instead of glucose, which produces ketones. The protein in meat is metabolized to form nitrogen waste, urea, and it's expelled in urine.

Ketosis can have very serious side effects like foul breath and urine. In addition, high concentrations of ketones have been known to cause comas. If you vary from an all-meat diet, even a smidgen, then the body converts back to processing carbohydrates, storing fat, and gaining weight. If you stay on the diet you basically ensure that you won't be healthy, so prepare your body for a series of complications. The meat diet will most likely promote inflammation and heavily tax the kidneys. Kidney problems generally go undetected until 90% of their function is lost. It is important to protect the kidneys because as we age, their ability to function is diminished. Also, colon complications may arise because of the lack of water and lack of mobility of the rotting putrid meat in your colon, which would be greatly facilitated by the addition of fruits, vegetables, water, and whole grains.

Mystery Diets

Flexible	★	Healthy	★	Maintainable	★	Satisfying	★

Mystery diets have mystifying logic to produce weight loss. One of the diets in this category includes the colors diet; it is based on food colors, which makes as much sense as eating foods based on the shape. The colors diet is based on a stop light. Red food—stop, do not eat. Yellow—warning, limit consumption. Green—go ahead, eat away. The intent of the diet is to encourage eating green vegetables. Although limiting red meat may be a good dietary decision, red vegetables have plenty of nutrients vital to a good diet.

Another mystifying diet is the blood type diet. Based on your blood type, different groups of foods are recommended while others are restricted. Despite blood type, everyone needs nutrients. If you like this diet, you might also be interested in the astrological diet.

Improving health is generally not the goal of mystery diets; they generally focus on promoting weight loss through obscure means. The body requires a cornucopia of nutrients and may soon grow weak and tired from the mystery menu. Mystery diets may be satisfying on a short-term basis, but not for very long. Mystery diets are quite inflexible; the food selections available are generally very limited, which may cease to be appealing very fast. Maintainability is another challenge of the mystery diets. The body is not a mystery machine; it requires a steady stream of nutrients minus toxins to promote weight loss.

Phase Diet

| Flexible | ★ | Healthy | ★ | Maintainable | ★ | Satisfying | ★ |

Some diets operate in phases; a phase to kick off the diet, a phase for the middle of the diet, and a phase to end the diet. The beginning phase is generally pretty tortuous with special rituals and little if any food. If you survive it, you'll be grateful for the water and sprouts provided during phase two. The last phase reintroduces you to a regular diet and may bring back all of the pounds you just lost.

Phase diets are generally not healthy and don't promote safe and lasting weight loss. During the dietary restrictions in the first phase, your metabolism may slow, hurting your weight loss efforts, not to mention depriving your body of the nutrients it needs to carry out everyday functions. It is vitally important to make wise dietary decisions to keep weight off, but most diets with phases do not take that into consideration.

Generally from the beginning to the end, phase diets are strictly regimented, not providing a smidgen of flexibility. Phase diets are not meant for the long haul; they are generally designed for a short period of time to maximize weight loss. While losing weight is great, to be successful a good diet must provide infinitely more.

Planned Meals and Packages

Flexible	★★	Healthy	★★	Maintainable	★★	Satisfying	★★

At times it is difficult to determine when to stop eating, especially when the food is good and there still more on the plate; that is one of the reasons prepackaged food has become a popular option. Prepackaged meals offer convenience and efficiency, while taking all of the guesswork out of eating. You don't have to wonder about the right amount because breakfast, lunch, and dinner is packed for you.

But there are downfalls associated with all shortcuts. Prepackaged meals are generally small, non-nutritive meals. Eating a small portion of a low-nutrient, high-calorie meal may help you lose weight, but you may still be hungry and it will do little, if anything, to improve your health. Prepackaged meals are the essence of unhealthiness; they are basically refined carbohydrates and meats, not fresh fruits and vegetables needed by the body to promote health. Some prepackaged plans do encourage adding fruits and vegetables. Prepackaged meals contain fewer calories, but about 25% of their calories are from fat. Not to mention, the meals are loaded with preservatives and other chemicals to increase their shelf life. Wouldn't you rather have a meal that is going to satisfy you and improve your health?

Prepackaged meals remove some of the responsibility of eating, but it is not realistic or feasible to eat prepackaged meals for the rest of your life. Prepackaged meals lack flexibility; you must be dependent on the planned meals morning, noon, and night. The show must go on and so must your diet. Prepackaged meal options are limited, which also limits the vitamins and nutrients delivered to your body; however, some prepackaged meals recommend vitamin supplements. Prepackaged meals can get expensive too, especially if you have to make meals for others. In addition, many people find it difficult to maintain the weight loss once they return to a regular diet.

Prepackaged meals help some people feel like they are not toiling through a diet because of the familiar foods; nonetheless, the portions are small. While some people are satisfied by limited portions, you may not be. Plain ole healthy eating provides more food while promoting your health and weight loss. You need a diet that is ready when you are, not some stifling prepackaged plan.

Prehistoric Diet

| Flexible | ★★ | Healthy | ★★★★ | Maintainable | ★★ | Satisfying | ★★★ |

The industrialization era created delectable refined foods with incredible taste and canned foods that extend the life of foods from days to years; however, while on the road to *wow* much of foods' nutritional value has been sacrificed.

With foods now deficient in nutrients, there is an increase in many diseases and illnesses, often called diseases of affluence, because many of the diseases common in industrialized countries are quite rare in unindustrialized countries.

Industrialization has become one of the scapegoats for the dismal state of health of many Americans, which has caused some to long for the simpler times of the long, long, long ago, like the diet enjoyed by the cavemen. However, making industrialization the scapegoat for the dismal state of health of millions is not the solution. It is neither realistic, nor necessary, to eat like a caveman for the rest of your life.

While the caveman diet does offer many unrefined fruits and vegetables, it eliminates all processed and refined foods. The caveman diet may be somewhat flexible and satisfying; however, most people want the best of both worlds, which may include healthy foods and a couple of tasty treats too. A diet should have nutrients to improve health while reducing the negative factors that will deteriorate your health.

Although there may be parts of the prehistoric diet that you can live with, you need a diet that you can accept wholeheartedly. Eating anything not part of the diet essentially means that you have abandoned the diet. No one is perfect and trying to achieve perfection can be frustrating.

Proportion Diet

Flexible	★★	Healthy	★	Maintainable	★	Satisfying	★★

Formulas are wonderful ideas. Formulas create full proof plans that anyone can follow successfully. This is part of the logic behind proportion diets. The body needs certain amount of nutrients daily so proportion diets regiment major categories of food each day to help ensure each category is not neglected, deficient, or overindulged.

For example, proportion diets may recommend eating a diet based on a proportion of foods like 30% proteins, 30% fats, and 40% carbs. In theory, the right proportion of protein, carbohydrates, and fats may sound good, but measuring food and configuring the right proportion of food may be difficult to determine for most people, may be an unnecessary expenditure of time, and may not provide sufficient nutrients.

All carbs, fats, and proteins are not created equal. Eating the right proportion of protein, carbs, and fat will not ensure a healthy diet. The three major categories of foods can be further dichotomized to identify the healthy and unhealthy categories. Besides, who wants to measure food all day? Diets shouldn't be so complicated. Either it's on the menu or it isn't. Proportions can be anything under the sun and that is just too obscure to promote good health and weight loss.

While proportion diets may be satisfying, it is an unnecessary expenditure of effort and time to calculate proportions for every meal. Besides, the body determines satiety, not calculations. Calculating proportions is just as tedious as calories counting; eat for nourishment, not to satisfy a formula.

Restriction Diet or Deprivation?

Flexible	★	Healthy	★	Maintainable	★	Satisfying	★

Many fad diets are restrictive; relying on limited food and nutrients to promote weight loss. Restricting your food is a way to lose weight; however, diets that limit, reduce, or restrict food can be tortuous. No matter how much you weigh, everyone gets hungry. Most restrictive diets promise a big upfront weight loss; however, usually the initial weight loss is water weight, and as soon as you eat anything remotely normal, the pounds roll right back again, and this time with a vengeance. There are tons of popular restrictive diets such as the cabbage, chocolate, cookie, fat, grapefruit, juice, and lemonade diets, which generally focus on a specific food, while restricting the gamut of foods needed to nourish the body.

The body is a quirky thing, sometimes it will immediately let you know that there is a problem, but sometimes it won't. Too much craziness and your body will go on strike, but hey, in your body's defense, it may have appeared that you didn't care or you'd have given it the nutrients needed.

Restrictive diets do not have much wiggle room. It is not feasible to hold your life hostage for a diet. Hunger can't be ignored; it can come on strong like a deep aching pang that will not subside until it is satisfied. It is no wonder why so many people fail on this type of diet. Diets that require physical pain are definitely not the solution. There is only so long that anyone can willingly starve. A diet must adjust to the ups, downs, and challenges of your life and a restrictive diet does not fit the bill. If a diet isn't sustainable, then it probably won't provide you with stellar results.

Diet concocters know there is not an iota of nutrition in restrictive diets, so they recommend supplements to provide nutrients; but why take supplements when you can have the real thing? Drop the zero nutrients diets, opt for health-building nutrients.

The body is complex and requires a series of micro- and macro-nutrients on a regular basis to carry out zillions of different functions. Limiting the body's nutrients reduces and even eliminates the body's ability to function. It is easier to stick with a plan if you are not fantasizing about the next meal.

Routine Diet

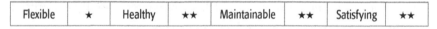

| Flexible | ★ | Healthy | ★★ | Maintainable | ★★ | Satisfying | ★★ |

Some diets recommend eating one food, day in and day out. Granted, eating a monotonous diet may avoid over-stimulating taste buds and overeating; however, a varied diet provides an array of beneficial nutrients that may not be successfully attained eating one food. There is not any single food that is able to provide all of the nutrients that the body needs; therefore, avoid diets that recommend eating the same food day in and day out like the plague.

The best diet has a cornucopia of different fruits and vegetables. Each fruit and vegetable has a different combination of vitamins and minerals working synergistically to enhance your health. If you decide to enjoy the same food for one meal—for instance, eating apples and oatmeal each morning for breakfast—it is important to ensure your other meals throughout the day provide additional nutrients to nourish your body.

Specialty Diet

Flexible	★	Healthy	★	Maintainable	★	Satisfying	★

Many people believe in the power of specialty diets because the diets seems so outrageous that something amazing has to result after following the diet, but most likely that is not the case. Generally, specialty diets are inflexible with a regimented menu of food. Like three parts rabbit toe, two parts honey, and one tooth of magical elf. As you might notice, specialty diet items are expensive and hard to find, which can be hard to maintain and worthless at helping you lose weight. Remember a variety of nutrients are needed to keep a well-functioning body.

The miniature morsels recommended by most specialty diets may leave your metabolism slowed and your body hungry and nutrient deprived. Diets with limited nutritional value recommend supplements, but they are a poor substitute for nutrient-rich foods. A diet that recommends popping pills to meet the nutritional requirements is not the right diet for anyone serious about making health improvements. Why follow a diet that is nutritionally void? Save yourself the extra trouble, select a nutrient-packed diet.

Gastric Surgery

Flexible	★	Healthy	★	Maintainable	★★	Satisfying	★

Having gastric surgery is a big decision. Although many gastric surgery patients have successfully lost significant amounts of weight, it is not a miraculous cure and success is not guaranteed. Surgery isn't the easy way out; it is a tool to help individuals that are in desperate need of losing weight.

Gastric surgery helps 90% of its patients lose 30 to 40% of their body weight within two years of having the surgery; however, weight loss is not automatic and some patients do regain the weight if a healthy lifestyle and good eating habits are not adopted. The stomach is quite elastic, and basically the surgery can be undone after three to five years. Unfortunately 20 to 35% of weight loss surgery patients regain their weight.

Surgery is not an option for everyone, or even individuals who are a little overweight. The cost of the surgery is pretty pricey at $40,000 to $50,000; however, some insurance companies will assist with the cost of the surgery, but certain conditions must be met like: a BMI of more than 40, health complications, documentation of lack of success with other methods, excessive weight not attributed to an endocrine disorder, no drug or alcohol abuse, willing to delay pregnancy, and a commitment to eating right and exercising. Before the surgery, patients generally endure a series of tests to ensure they are physically and psychologically fit. Talking to someone who has actually had the surgery and lived with the changes is highly recommended for those individuals interested in the surgery.

There are multiple types of gastric surgery available. Adjustable gastric banding (AGB) reduces the area of the stomach with an adjustable band that can be tightened or loosened. Vertical banded gastroplasty (VBG) reduces the area of the stomach with staples. This type of surgery has been found to be more successful than the AGB; however, for many the success is short term.

The biliopancreatic diversion (BPD) and the roux-en-Y are two types of gastric bypasses that are routinely done to promote weight loss. The biliopancreatic diversion reduces the size of the stomach and attaches it to the last part of the small intestines to avoid food absorption. The roux-en-Y is the gastric bypass procedure most commonly performed in the US. The stomach is restricted, while part of the intestines is removed to reduce the body's ability to absorb nutrients. Malabsorptive weight loss surgery is successful because you don't store calories you can't absorb.

Gastric surgeons use traditional and laparoscopic incisions to perform the surgery. A traditional open surgery uses an incision of six to eight inches versus laparoscopic surgery that uses a tiny incision. Although multiple factors contribute to the healing process, laparoscopic incisions generally heal within two weeks, versus traditional surgery, which may require four weeks to heal.

It's not just surgery and then you're happy and super-skinny. It is a long hard road that may not end with success. Patients who endure gastric bypass permanently change the way that the body operates, and the changes are irreversible. The changes do not promote optimal performance or health, but rather decrease it.

After the gastric surgery, there may be complications and a series of generally unwanted side effects that may be life-long factors, which include, but are not limited to: abdominal pain, carbohydrate intolerance, constipation, dehydration, diarrhea, fouler-smelling stool, hair loss, heartburn, malnutrition, muscle loss, protein intolerance, vomiting, and organ leakage into the abdominal cavity. Phew! Not to mention, gallstones are frequently formed with rapid weight loss; therefore, as an added bonus gallbladders are frequently removed during gastric surgeries.

Vigilant diet control is even more crucial after gastric surgery because the stomach is elastic and weight gain may occur without dietary caution, which may cause serious side effects. After gastric surgery, desperately needed nutrients are often not absorbed. Weight loss surgery patients must take supplements to provide adequate nutrition to compensate for the negative effects of the surgery. Iron and B_{12} deficiencies occur in more than 30% of patients. Some patients develop malnutrition from the inability to absorb vitamins and nutrients, which may result in health complications. Many patients cannot tolerate the foods they used to enjoy. Plus, the surgery drastically reduces the stomach size so a meal may be as small as a spoonful to a cupful, which requires eating tiny meals throughout the day for sufficient nourishment. Liquids reduce the amount of food consumed during a meal and may be better tolerated before or after meals.

Dumping syndrome also known as rapid gastric emptying is another one of the many side effects of gastric surgery. Dumping can occur immediately or up to three hours after eating and is caused by food rapidly dumping from the stomach to the small intestines, which can cause anal leakage, cramps, and nausea, as well as varying degrees of discomfort. As a result of dumping, individuals may experience an aversion to eating, which may promote weight loss and malnutrition. Adequate nutrients, no liquid with meals, reduced sugar, reduced citrus, reduced fried food, smaller portions, and limited movement after eating may reduce the dumping syndrome.

A smaller pouch is easier to fill and may produce a feeling of satiety and fullness, but really how satisfying can it be to eat a cupful or couple of spoonful of foods? The flexibility to eat a wide variety of foods is eliminated after gastric surgery. Eating becomes a calculated and deliberate process. Gastric bypass is a last ditch effort to help people who desperately need to lose weight to improve their health. Overtime, the surgical alterations may not endure and emergency surgery may be required to fix leakages. Scar tissue from the surgery may cause additional complications and require additional surgery as well.

Fasting and Detoxifying

Flexible	★	Healthy	★	Maintainable	★	Satisfying	★

"I saw few die of hunger; of eating, a hundred thousand."
— Benjamin Franklin

"He that eats till he is sick must fast till he is well."
— Thomas Fuller (1654-1734). Letter to
Samuel Johnson, 13 September 1750.

The diets du jour like fasting and detoxifying have conjured a lot of interest. Detox diets operate on the premise that the body must be detoxified. There are tons of claims that fasting will cleanse, detoxify, and purge all of the putrid garbage consumed and absorbed from a regular diet and toxic environment, which sounds great and considering what we put in our bodies, it seems necessary.

While a fast may be good under limited circumstances, it is important to remember that a fast is a restrictive diet, which doesn't provide your body with the nutrients needed in order to carry out vital bodily functions. In addition, when you don't eat you may grow weak from the lack of nutrition, get headaches, slow your metabolism, or even worse, become gravely ill from the lack of nutrition and weakened immune system.

Although some people think that they are helping their body eliminate the accumulated garbage in the colon, fasting is not the best way to accomplish this goal. In fact, fasting may actually hurt the body more than junk food. If you really want to help detoxify your body, it starts with feeding, not starving your body.

When fasting, beyond being hungry, you are depriving your body of the essential nutrients it needs for survival. Although the body is able to store some vitamins and minerals, it still needs a daily supply of nutrients. Fasting may cause your body to steal nutrients from another source within the body, skip vital functions, or a fate even worse. The worst part is you may not notice the damage until later, which may complicate the diagnosis process. Good nutrition helps ward off disease and sickness.

The body is a pretty smart little gizmo; when it catches on that you are not taking in any food, it will likely slow down your metabolism to conserve energy. So instead of burning your normal amount of calories, you may burn hundreds less calories per day, which may significantly thwart your plans to lose weight. In addition, you may be more tired and lethargic without adequate nutrition. That's the worst combination ever—no food and a slow metabolism. ☹

Many foods that are currently enjoyed are virtually devoid of any nutritional value and damage the body; foods like natural and artificial sweeteners, meats, processed and refined food, and saturated and trans-fats. Additionally, we come into contact and even ingest many toxins from chemicals, herbicides, and pesticides, which overwhelm many of the body's organs like the kidneys, liver, lungs, and skin. Granted excess weight and toxins strain the body; however, what took years to accumulate can't be undone in one day, one week, or even a month.

Some people think fasting provides the body's many organs a well-deserved hiatus by reducing food, but it is not necessary. Fortunately the body works 24/7, never needing a break. The body's organs are not kindergartners whining for a nap—their most important requirement is good nutrition. Just think of the body as a self-cleaning oven. You supply the right materials and the body does the rest. The body was designed to digest food to extract energy and nutrients. Forgoing food may give the body some rest, but it may also cause more harm than good.

Many people already reap the rewards of fasting every day; it's called sleep. Considering that the body has a fast daily, additional fasts are simply redundant. If you want to intensify your fast don't eat after a certain hour every night, thus giving your body the time that it needs to rejuvenate. In the morning, break the fast with breakfast.

While this diet is pretty easy to maintain, basically just water and go; the difficulty lies in the hunger that persists. Temptation is at every step—hey when you're deprived, even dirt may start to look good. Fasting does not offer much flexibility, it basically eliminates most forms of sustenance, which may be challenging to endure. You can even feel the body's dissatisfaction with the grumbling and moaning in your tummy.

Non-surgical Gastric Shrinking

| Flexible | ★ | Healthy | ★ | Maintainable | ★ | Satisfying | ★ |

People want to eat until they are full and satiated, it's just a natural thing to do. The optimal goal is to satisfy hunger, not to eat until you are full. Portion sizes are out of control and generally much more food is provided. When the food is present, many people eat a significantly greater amount of food than is needed to fulfill energy and nutritional requirements. Overeating gigantisizes the stomach to accommodate more and more food. The quantity a stomach can hold varies from person to person, it can be as small as a change purse holding a couple of ounces or as large as a tank holding over 100 ounces. After a significant period of overeating, the stomach may become a bottomless pit requiring trough loads to become full. Professional competitive eaters don't just show up one day hoping to eat more than their competitors, nor do they sit at home for weeks leading up to the big competition, refraining from food and hoping that they'll be so hungry that they will eat faster and more than everyone else. They are busy training. Training is essentially eating more and more to expand the stomach. In essence, many Americans are professional eaters; going day in and day out, taking advantage of all the meal deals, stretching and upsizing their once fist-sized stomachs to watermelon proportions.

A lifetime of eating until you are full may have negative side effects on your waistline. But just as the stomach was expanded it can be shrunken, albeit it's not as much fun. Shrinking the size of the stomach can be done slowly by reducing the amount of food consumed at each meal. A smaller stomach is not going to happen overnight, but it will definitely help you reach your weight goals if you stick with it. It may seem difficult at first, but may become easier over time.

As important as reducing the amount of food consumed at each meal, it's also important to reduce the amount of liquid that is consumed. Supersized alcoholic beverages, coffees, sodas, and sugary fruity concoctions can pack a lot of calories. Excessive liquids can also increase the size of the stomach.

There are other and perhaps better alternatives than fasting, but it can assist you in making some important changes within your body. For some people, fasting may be a good alternative to gastric surgery. As an added bonus, you will not permanently mutilate the insides of your body. Fasting can be used as a tool to help you reach your weight loss goals; however, it is not the cure or the only necessary step. In addition to promoting weight loss, fasting may help one to purge cravings and bad eating habits by cleansing the body and the palate. Learning the feeling of true hunger can help you differentiate cravings and hunger and may strengthen your resolve.

The gastric shrinking road is somewhat like the road travelled by gastric surgery patients. Both are excruciating, but for different reasons. Of course, having your insides cut up wins the debate over most painful, but limiting your food to shrink your stomach is no cake walk either. Fasting helps the stomach, an elastic organ, to shrink, shrink, shrink to a smaller size. A smaller stomach fills faster, which is essentially the same concept as gastric surgery without all of the slicing and dicing. You could have someone cut you open and permanently muck up your insides or you could shrink your stomach yourself through fasting.

Most people at one point or another have shrunk or expanded their stomachs. Stomach shrinking may be less common than the expanding, but think back to the last time that you were sick. Really, really, barfing into the toilet, bile-puking sick. Are you there yet? While on the road to recovery you may remember eating little bites or two and presto, you were full.

Fasting can be very strenuous and demanding and is not recommended for everyone. If you have any special health concerns fasting should be avoided. Some of the special health concerns include, but are not limited to:

Children	Hypoglycemic	Nursing moms
Diabetics	Ill	Pregnant women
Elderly	Medication consumers	Underweight

There are many types and variations of fasts. Mono-diets include one type of food throughout day; to liquitarianism, where a variety of liquids like broth, nut milks, tea, and water are consumed. A juice fast, as the name implies, includes only juice. But it does not mean that you can have more juice to make up the difference between a regular meal and just juice. A regular serving of juice is eight to sixteen ounces. Fresh juice is packed with vitamins and minerals that your body will enjoy, but it is also concentrated—all the nutritious fiber has been removed and only the sweet and highly caloric juice is left.

Due to the intense nature of fasting, there are things that you should do before, during, and after the fast to help you maximize your efforts. While adequate hydration is extremely important during a fast, beverages like alcohol, carbonated drinks, and coffee should be avoided. Water is the best choice; it facilitates many important functions within the body like flushing out toxins and promoting healing.

A fast can range anywhere from a day to as long as you can withstand it, but generally they are not recommended for more than 30 days. Fasts can also vary from abstinence from eating, skipping a meal, fasting every other day, or fasting one day a week.

Some fasts may be broken up into several phases like: the pre-fast, fast, and after-fast. Each phase helps the body transition. Before a fast, don't consume a lot of food to sustain you through the fast. In fact, a fast usually begins with a pre-fast to help the body adjust. The first days of the fast are generally the toughest. After the first couple of days on the fast, hunger should dissipate and the rest of the fast should be easier. Although it may be initially difficult, it is important to try to persevere through the fast to arrive at the other side with a smaller stomach.

The pre-fast can be implemented gradually to reduce the stress on the body and help the body adjust. A pre-fast may last from one to three days to help you transition from solids to liquids. Pre-fast foods include fruits and vegetables, preferably raw, to prepare the body for the fast. While vegetables are recommended as a pre-fast food, nightshade vegetables like eggplant, green peppers, potatoes and tomatoes may irritate the stomach and should be avoided. Other foods to avoid include dairy, fish, grains, and meat. It is important to not contaminate your body during the fast. Eating foods that are not a part of the fast can significantly reduce the progress achieved.

Even though you are trying to lose weight, your body still needs nutrients. Therefore, the best fasts include fruits and vegetables. Fruits and vegetables have most of the vitamins and minerals the body needs daily and they can help absorb toxins. If needed, supplements may provide additional nutrients your body requires.

To successfully maintain a fast, refrain from temptation. Don't visit places that will torture you with visual and olfactory temptations. It is important to focus on other things besides eating. The fast won't last forever. And after you're finished you should be able to enjoy smaller portions satisfactorily.

Try not to schedule your fast around social events or during strenuous activity. The body consumes less energy during a fast; therefore, it is important to conserve energy. However, some forms of exercise are recommended like: biking, dancing swimming, and walking. In addition, warm temperatures are better suited for fasting.

You may also notice a significant reduction in your bowel movements: little in, little out. Stored toxins may be released and circulated through the system to be purged. On the way out of the body, toxins may cause a series of side effects known as healing events or healing crises like cramping, depression, headache, nausea, stomach pain, and weakness.

You can have a planned end point or you can resume eating when strong urges to eat return. The length at which a fast can be endured is different for everyone. Most fasts can be endured safely for seven days or as long as 30 days.

Fasting Healing Events		
Acne	Faintness	Muscle aches
Asthma	Fatigue	Nausea
Bad breath	Fever	Rash
Bronchitis	Headaches	Runny nose
Diarrhea	Hot flashes	Stuffy nose
Dizziness	Irregular heartbeat	Weakness
Eczema	Irregular menstruation	

At the end of the fast it is important not to overindulge. Gradually add solid foods starting with fruits and vegetables, while abstaining from refined carbohydrates and meats. Consuming an unrestricted diet immediately after a fast may cause negative side effects.

Gastric bypass and non-surgical gastric shrinking are tools to help promote weight loss, but neither are 100% guaranteed. Unlike the after-effects of gastric surgery you will not lose your appetite based on infections, nausea, pain, and sickness. Nor will you have warning signs of dumping after eating too much. Be careful, eating tyrannosaurus rex portions eliminates any progress that you achieve. Just as the stomach can shrink, it can expand.

Vegetarianism

Flexible	★	Healthy	★	Maintainable	★	Satisfying	★

Being a vegetarian is not a guarantee that you will lose weight or improve your health; excessive eating, too much fat, refined carbs, and poor lifestyle choices can cause a vegetarian to experience health and weight issues as well.

There are multiple forms of vegetarianism. Some would say either you are or you aren't, but this is not the case for flexitarians or semi-vegetarians who are primarily vegetarians, but enjoy meat every blue moon.

Lacto-ovo or ovo-lacto vegetarians generally abstain from meat while enjoying dairy products and eggs. Adding diary and eggs to the diet provides essential nutrients not included in a strictly plant product diet. Pescatarians are vegetarians who avoid land animals, while enjoying the nutrients provided by seafood.

Vegans on the other hand, eat strictly a plant product diet, thereby abstaining from any animal products or foods that may be contaminated by animal products. Raw vegans take veganism a step further and refrain from foods that have been cooked at temperatures higher than 115° F. Avoiding cooked foods helps maintain the nutrients packed in food while avoiding the negative by-products that may be produced from cooking foods.

A macrobiotic diet is the ultimate vegan diet consisting of unprocessed fruits, vegetables, and whole grains. The macrobiotic diet emphasizes nutrient rich Asian vegetables like daikon and seaweed while excluding inflammatory foods like refined and processed carbohydrates.

A vegetarian diet provides a fair amount of flexibility, everything except meat; but there are new discoveries every day and there may be additional unknown benefits contained in meat. Meat is an important part of the diet that provides good sources of iron, zinc, and B_{12}. Animals are the only source of B_{12}; therefore, vegetarians should consume foods that have been enriched with B_{12}. Although plant products provide many needed vitamins and minerals, often they do not contain sufficient levels or balanced ratios. Vegetarians should be diligent to ensure their diets contain adequate amounts of calcium, iron, vitamin D, and zinc.

While a vegetarian diet can be satisfying, meat is a well-loved food and going without meat for the rest of your life may be a difficult task. Therefore, it may be necessary to weigh the actual benefits in light of what you are giving up to what you are actually gaining. The best of both worlds is reducing meat while increasing fruits and vegetables. If your diet feels incomplete, it may be your body's cry for help. Satisfaction will help you stick with your diet.

At first thought, a vegetarian diet may seem very healthy, but a vegetarian diet can be just as unhealthy as any other diet if refined and processed carbohydrates are the main component. To get the most benefits from a vegetarian diet it is important to have plenty of unrefined and fruits and vegetables.

Four Stars Diet ★ How to Make Your Diet Work

| Flexible | ★★★★ | Healthy | ★★★★ | Maintainable | ★★★★ | Satisfying | ★★★★ |

> *"People are so worried about what they eat between Christmas and the New Year, but they really should be worried about what they eat between the New Year and Christmas."*
> — UNKNOWN

Weight goes on so effortlessly, yet every minute of dieting is generally torture. Let's face it; no one can live on diet forever, for most of us, not even a short while. Every moment on a diet becomes seemingly unbearable. The memories of savory, delectable goodies emerge so strongly that just the thought of not having them creates cravings the size of mountains. So what do you do? Wait painstakingly until your diet ends in two weeks then gorge yourself? Break your diet and have the goodies? Or simply deny yourself the treats you want most?

For many, the mere mention of the word "diet" brings back flashbacks and nightmares of starvation, but not this time. It is not the end of the world just because you have decided to modify the way that you eat; in fact, it's a whole new world. With time, it will energize you.

What would you do to lose weight? Spend money, pop pills, try a crazy fad diet? Many people are willing to try everything but the steps that will work. Sometimes, the solution seems too plain, too trite, too basic to provide results. Many people think major weight loss must come from some mysterious and magical source like a potion, pill, mumbo jumbo, or elective surgery that connects the stootum to the dootum, and then shoot everything out the tootum; but actually it isn't that complicated. Why is it so easy to trust the complex and the extraordinary, instead of the basic reality?

Each person has specific factors contributing to his or her health and weight like level of physical activity, genetics, metabolism, and diet. Everyone is different; we are not one size, nor are diets. Two people can eat the exact same meal, while one loses weight and the other gains weight.

Following a diet may not lead you to success, even if you follow the secret diet ritual precisely. Not to mention, following a precise eating plan is difficult for most people. The truth is most diets don't work; even when we follow the diet's directions enduring hunger, pain, and torture—pounds stay put. Why should someone else's diet work for you? Your diet should be tailored to you.

The best cures and health maintenance rely on the food we eat, but sooner rather than later is the key. Time is of the essence. Miracles may not happen overnight, but they do happen. Don't rely on the fallible and imperfect drugs and surgeries to slim your waist. Take preemptive action by improving your diet, which may not only improve your health, but save money toward insurance and medical costs.

There is a need to improve the way that many people think of and consume food. Although food gives you the energy to stay alive, unhealthy food robs you of a healthy life and precious years to come. A diet does not just include that horrible event that causes you hunger, sacrifice, and starvation until you get to your desired weight or physique; a diet is your everyday choices that supplies you with energy and nourishment; however, not all food is nourishing. In fact, some foods are downright dangerous.

Some say ignorance is bliss; but it may kill you slowly day by day, which doesn't sound like much bliss. It is important to learn about food to make the best decisions for yourself in any situation. By learning more about your diet you can effortlessly make better choices for yourself on a daily basis to ensure that you are doing all that you can to promote your health and weight loss. Learning how food affects your weight and health can be very liberating.

Many people have no knowledge of the true effect of lifestyle and food on their body. It is in your best interest to be armed with the information that can help you make better decisions for your health and diet. Knowing more about the effects of your diet on your health will help you make better decisions. The upcoming chapters will armor your with the knowledge needed to face the daily battle of eating.

The diet that many Americans routinely enjoy is laden with many landmines that routinely promote disease and inflammation, which endangers health and longevity. A diet should not make you sick or cause ridiculous side effects. Nutrition-related illnesses lead to more deaths than environmental factors like pollution and smoking.

It is not enough to simply rely on calorimeters, guidelines, packaged meals, and others tactics to lose weight. You have to learn the best ways to eat and nourish yourself. There is not one diet that can help you tackle the daily temptations and unexpected challenges like your knowledge. It is not feasible to live on a crazy restricted diet for the rest of your life, nor is it necessary. What is necessary? The knowledge of food and how it will affect your health and weight. This knowledge will empower you to make good decisions in any situation to help manage your weight and improve your health. Diets du jour and fads will come and go, but your knowledge will not forsake you.

Research shows that the most successful diets are low maintenance, not the diets with strict regimens that require a calorimeter, food scale, or a stop watch. Besides, who wants to be hassled by the restrictions and convictions of a diet. Don't eat this; eat a morsel of that. Strict regimens are too much work.

Making dietary changes can be easy when you understand the effect various foods will have on your health and weight. You don't have to eliminate anything out of your diet. You may continue to eat the foods that you enjoy, but some reductions and additions of nutritious food may create vast improvements. You can eat what makes sense for you and your diet. The goal is to make better decisions for yourself. With little modifications, you can sculpt a diet that will promote a healthy weight and body.

Your diet must be nutritious to promote your health. Of course the goal is to lose weight, but if your body is not running optimally and getting the nutrients it needs, you may never reach your weight loss goals. To be successful, diets must take care of the whole body. That means your body can't be starved. When nutrients are missing, disease may develop. Many fad diets fail to properly nourish the body, which may thwart weight loss efforts. One of the most important things that you can do to lose weight is eating healthy foods to reduce inflammation and nourish your body.

A diet must be easily maintainable, even under the toughest conditions. Life is hectic enough. A diet should not be an added source of stress; it should be a life enhancement. A diet should help you meet the challenges ahead, not be the challenge ahead.

Diets have to be flexible to coordinate with schedules, moods, and emergencies of life. Flexibility provides infinite choices, not limits choices. You live and eat in the real world, you need real food options. You can't go off in the middle of the day searching for the whisker of an Irish leprechaun just because a diet says that it is crucial to your weight loss. The only way that crazy items may help you lose weight is through burning calories on a long wild goose chase.

A diet is only good if it works for you; it could be the best diet in the world for someone else, but if it's not a good fit, then it won't work. To be successful you should develop a collective understanding of food and its effect on the body, then pick and choose the elements that best fit your goals, lifestyle, preferences, and motivation to develop Your Diet. We base decisions on our knowledge, but when our knowledge increases we can do infinitely more for ourselves. The best part is, it's not a diet in the silly restrictive "I can't eat anything" sense of the word, but a maintainable regimen that promotes health, satisfaction, and weight loss.

Why do diets always want you to change for them? This time your diet is going to change for you. Now that you have seen diets that won't work, it is time to learn what will. With increased knowledge of food, you will be able to craft a diet that will work for you. This diet will be entirely your creation. The upcoming chapters will provide you with information that will help your sculpt a satisfying diet that will be easily maintainable, healthy, satisfying, and flexible.

Why will this diet work, when others won't? Because you have the formula on how food will affect your body. The information the upcoming chapters will help you craft Your Diet; this information will be with you 24/7 to help you make the best dietary decisions to help the pounds roll off. This knowledge will influence your eating decisions and impact the way that you manage food and life to create sustainable weight loss. This diet will work because it is flexible, healthy, maintainable, and satisfying.

PART II

What You Should Know Before You Take Another Bite

Plant Products 5

"Let thy food be they medicine, and let thy medicine be thy food."
— Hippocrates

Junk Food

*"Those who think they have no time for healthy eating
will sooner or later have to find time for illness."*
— MODIFIED FROM: EDWARD STANLEY (1826–1893)
FROM THE CONDUCT OF LIFE

CARBS, CARBS, CARBS! They're everywhere—low carbs, no carbs. What's the deal? Are they really evil? Like cars run on gasoline, the human body needs carbohydrates to run efficiently and effectively. Carbohydrates break down into glucose, which is ushered to cells to be used as a source of energy. Some cars can run on alternative fuels, but they generally won't get you as far as the good stuff. Same concept with carbs, sometimes the garbage maybe a little cheaper and may even taste better, but it's not going to get you very far or do much for your body.

Carbohydrates are essential to a good diet; however, all carbs are not created equal. It is vital to choose carbohydrates that optimize your diet. Carbohydrates include complex carbohydrates, simple carbohydrates, and dietary fiber. Simple and complex carbohydrates differ in the units of sugar they contain. Simple carbohydrates have one or two units of sugar, which are easy for the body to break down and digest.

Simple carbohydrates are only part of the story. Unlike simple carbohydrates, complex carbohydrates have long complicated chains of sugar, and depending on the starch, they may be more difficult to break down and digest, which may delay the release of glucose, reduce the impact of sugar on the blood, and provide a longer feeling of fullness. Complex carbs include starches and fibers like beans, brown rice, corn, potatoes, and wheat.

Simple carbohydrates include refined and unrefined carbohydrates. Some refined carbohydrates seem perfectly harmless, even good, but a closer look may reveal some hidden perils that may impede efforts to improve your health. Refining and processing increases shelf life, reduces food-related illnesses, enhances texture and flavor, but decreases nutritional value. Refined carbs are notorious empty calorie foods; they are stripped of their nutritional content through processing and refining, leaving just the bare elements. Refined foods provide tons of taste and calories while your body reaps none of the benefits it expects from food.

When selecting foods, be on the lookout for foods void of any nutritional value. This does not mean that you can never enjoy refined carbs; however, the quantity and the frequency should be thoughtfully considered before you eat them. Limit calories from refined carbohydrates like alcohol, bread, cookies, pastas, sugars, white flour, and white rice. Subsisting on a diet filled with cooked, processed, and refined food does not provide the body with sufficient nutrients. A body without the required vitamins, minerals, and nutrients may succumb to a series of diseases, health complications, and malnourishment.

The refining process leaves carbohydrates so devoid of any nutritional value that food manufacturers try to enrich refined foods with a couple of vitamins and minerals, but it is a sore attempt to replace all of the nutritious elements removed. B vitamins, iron, and other essential minerals are routinely added to bread to replace some of the nutrients.

Refined carbs may satisfy hunger, but not for very long. Refined and processed foods may promote hunger because the body has not received sufficient nutrients and is unsatisfied. Poor nutrition creates a gnawing urge to eat immediately after eating. If you're still hungry right after you eat, evaluate the nutritional content of your last meal. Was it nutritious? Did it provide your body with the nutrients needed?

Low blood sugar triggers hunger and cravings. The brain requires a steady stream of energy throughout the day. Simple and refined carbohydrates are easily broken down, digested, and generally raise glucose levels quickly. Refined foods are the body's obvious choice for a snack because they taste good and the body loves sources of easily digested energy. Not to mention that sweet foods make your body feel good by releasing endorphins, the body's natural painkiller.

Although they satisfy hunger, refined carbohydrates increase glucose levels. When high glucose levels are detected, the pancreas immediately responds with the release of insulin. However, two to four hours after eating low quality carbs like refined carbohydrates, blood sugar plummets, creating hypoglycemic symptoms like headaches, hunger attacks, and mood swings. Excess body fat requires additional insulin to stabilize blood sugar. Over time, increased weight and intake of refined foods taxes the pancreas and promotes the development of diabetes.

Fruits and Vegetables

"The road to health is paved with vegetables,
fruits, beans, rice, and grains."
— POLLY STRAND. LETTER TO SAN FRANCISCO
CHRONICLE, 19 MARCH 1993.

I don't like them and I won't eat them. Yep, sometimes we hold fast to our beliefs. We didn't like vegetables as kids and we don't like them as adults; but you've changed, and so have your taste buds. Most children have significantly more taste buds than adults. The highly refined and sensitive taste buds of children are a built-in safety mechanism. Children don't always have the knowledge to determine what foods are safe to eat, so their taste buds are ultra-sensitive to bitter and sour foods that may be poisonous while sweet foods generally are safer. Unfortunately, some nutritious foods fall into the bitter, unsavory category. But as our age and knowledge increases, the acuity of the built-in safety mechanism fades, allowing adults to enjoy a wider range of foods. Vegetables should taste better than when you were a kid, so throw away the memories of what's yucky and rediscover food.

Fruits and vegetables may be more expensive, even more expensive out of season, not as convenient as packaged carbs, and not laden with a ton of chemicals that give an extraordinary sensational taste. So you'll give up a few things, but you'll gain much more. For the few cons they present, fruits and vegetables present significant benefits.

It may be cheaper and faster to pop open a bag of refined carbs, but fruits and vegetables are well worth the added expense and effort. You get what you pay for, and either way you go, you'll pay now or later. If you don't put forth the effort, you're not going to get improvements. Fruits and vegetables pack powerful punches that nourish and heal your body.

If you think that eating healthy is expensive, what price are you willing to pay for your health? To reduce the risk of cancer, diabetes, heart disease, stroke, and other chronic illnesses that can take your life? What price would you pay to avoid relying on daily medications that slowly kill you while keeping you alive?

A good diet can help you achieve your desired weight, but it is also pivotal in helping you achieve good health. Many doctors have witnessed significant health improvements in individuals who eat primarily plant products, even more significant improvements than drugs and surgery. This is not to say that plant products are the panacea of health; however, many research studies show positive results from eating a diet that includes fruits, vegetables, and whole grains. Furthermore, studies have found that people who regularly eat plant products are less likely to get cancer and coronary diseases. Plant product diets also improve the body's ability to burn calories, rather than depositing fat on the body.

Plant products contain most of the nutrients that the body needs, like essential fatty acids, fiber, minerals, nutrients, phytochemicals, and protein to promote health. Fruits and vegetables have the ability to:

+ Enhance the diet
+ Reduce blood pressure
+ Prevent memory failure
+ Promote weight management
+ Reduce gastrointestinal complications
+ Reduce the risk of cardiac complications
+ Protect against cataracts and macular degeneration

The storehouse of vitamins, minerals, and nutrients in fruits and vegetables serve to diminish and eliminate the effect of many diseases. Some of the amazing disease fighters include, but are not limited to: allum compounds, beta carotene, dithiolthiones, fiber, flavonoids, folic acid, idole-3-carbinol, inositol hexaphosphate, isoflavones, isothiocyanates, luetin, lycopene, phytosterols, protease inhibitors, and selenium.

Phytonutrients are chemicals produced only by plants present in a variety of foods including beans, fruits, grains, and vegetables. Approximately 5,000 phytochemicals have been identified; however, it is estimated that countless more have not been identified. Phytonutrients include antioxidants, glyconutrients, minerals, and vitamins. The most well-known phytonutrients include carotenoids and fiber. Phytochemicals vividly color fruits and vegetables. Luetin makes yellows, lycopene makes red, carotenes makes oranges, anthicyanin makes blues, and still others like vitamin C and E are colorless. Phytonutrients provide numerous health benefits like facilitating digestion, maintaining cellular health, preventing carcinogens, and reducing cholesterol. Phytochemicals create a resistance to disease, repair DNA, detoxify the body, strengthen the immune system, and create treatments against cancer, cardiovascular, and other health complications. Numerous dietary studies have been conducted and generally they all conclude that fruits and vegetables are the best foods for the body.

The antioxidants within fruits and vegetables have been shown in numerous research studies to reduce and or eliminate the likelihood of developing various diseases. The profound benefits of antioxidants have prompted scientists to isolate them from fruits and vegetables in an attempt to replicate and magnify their valuable effects on the body. Through studies, researchers have learned that while antioxidant extracts may provide some benefits to the consumer, they do not pack the intensity or the effectiveness found in unrefined fruits or vegetables. Therefore, don't be persuaded to substitute your daily orange or grapes for a supplement that claims to pack the same punch; it is most likely not possible.

Fruits are the perfect snack and they offer a fountain of benefits. Eating fruits and vegetables not only satisfies hunger, but provide nutrients and fiber. Unlike prepackaged snacks, fruits and vegetables are not loaded with chemicals and preservatives. There are many ways to incorporate vegetables into your diet like:

+ Drink green smoothies
+ Eat a salad at each meal
+ Snack on raw vegetables
+ Mix or blend vegetables in meals

+ Stuff sandwiches with vegetables
+ Eat steamed vegetables with dinner

Diary, meats, and oils are packed with so many calories it's difficult to eat them without ingesting excess calories. This is not a problem when eating fruits and vegetables. Vegetables contain a lot of water and are a good source of fiber, minerals, and vitamins, and they have virtually no fat. Aside from avocados that are packed with good oils, most vegetables are fat free. Without condiments, most fruits have less than 60 calories per half cup and vegetables have 25 calories per half cup.

Unlike drugs, medications, and supplements, fruits and vegetables are nontoxic at high dosage. They provide a storehouse of vitamins and minerals, without the dangerous side effects. But as a word of caution, an overdose of carrots can give you an orange pallor; while too much beet juice can darken urine and poop. Although some fruits are acidic, you don't have to worry about them contributing to acidic conditions within the body because they are dominated by their alkalizing minerals and salts.

Fruits and vegetables can have a tremendous healing effect on the body. There are countless stories of individuals that have found cures nothing short of a miracle, simply by adding fruits and veggies to their diets. Fruits and vegetables have many phytochemicals that can heal the body. Vitamin supplements attempt to replicate the beneficial effects of phytochemicals; but as scientists have discovered, individual isolated phytochemicals do not have the power of whole unrefined fruits and vegetables.

The results of a research study shows that individuals who consumed natural carotenoids had more than 40% less macular degenerative disease. The eye disease cataracts has been found to affect half of Americans over the age of 80; however, individuals who consume the antioxidant luetin found in spinach were 50% less likely to develop cataracts.

Another research study shows that individuals who consumed at least five servings of greens per week had 88% less disease than those who didn't. There are many scientific studies that show a clear relationship with low fruit consumption and digestive, bladder, and prostate cancer. Researchers have found that diets rich in fruits and vegetables while low in meat have lower instances of colon cancer. By simply increasing the amount of fruits and vegetables consumed daily, individuals can significantly reduce their risk for colorectal cancer. Eating fruits and vegetables not only promotes a healthy weight, but research results show that by eating three servings of fruits a day will decrease the risk of a stroke by more than 20%. Longevity studies all report that fruits and vegetables improve health and extend life.

Fruits and vegetables not only improve internal body conditions, but external body conditions as well. Many people notice after adding fruits and vegetables to their diet, there are significant improvements to the condition and the appearance of the skin—causing a reduction or elimination of acne, rashes, and skin growths.

We all know that change can be scary, but it also can be wonderfully fantastic. Instead of thinking about all of the things that you are going to give up, think about all of the foods you will add to your diet. Modifying your diet may initially be a major adjustment, but after a short period of time your body will adjust and learn to like, even love, the improvements. You'll love the way that you look, the way that you feel, the increased energy, and new pleasures that you experience. And by improving your food selections, you may be able to eat more food than you did before because now the food has more nutrients and fewer calories. In addition, the cooking style may completely change your opinion of the food, whether it is baked, grilled, raw, sautéed, or steamed. The addition of a few herbs and spices can enhance the flavor even more.

Like any new relationship, you have to give it a chance. You may not like every fruit or vegetable, but with a reasonable opportunity, a love of new foods will grow. So give new foods a little time, seasoning, and a chance.

What you eat is more important than how much you eat. Most Americans are overfed, yet undernourished. The typical American diet is severely lacking in fiber, fruits, and vegetables. Less than 10% of Americans consume the daily recommendation of five fruits and vegetables. Dietary studies show that almost 90% of people in the US don't consume the recommended amount of vitamin C. Due to tricky advertising and gimmicks, many Americans believe that they can slyly get their nutrition from fruit juices, vitamins, and processed foods that have limited nutritional value, but this is not true.

A variety of fruits and vegetables is the best way to get all of the nutrients needed to promote health. Five to ten fruits and vegetables per day are recommended to provide the fiber and the nutrients the body needs to be healthy and well. Although five to ten may seem like a lot, it could be a lot less than you think.

One serving of a fruit or vegetable:
+ One cup uncooked
+ Half cup or 4 oz. cooked

There are pros and cons with everything, even with fruits and vegetables. Potatoes and tomatoes are some of the most highly consumed fruits and vegetables eaten in the US thanks to French fries and ketchup, but their categorization as a fruit or vegetable is baffling. Ketchup is highly processed and refined, barely resembling the round red balls of nutrients that grow from vines. While potatoes are another highly consumed vegetable, they're generally fried or paired with very unhealthy condiments. While potatoes and tomatoes are plant products, if they are demonized by processing or unsavory elements they shouldn't be counted as part of your five fruits and vegetables.

In order to reap the benefits of eating fruits and vegetables, don't fry them in oil, refine them, or add chemicals to them.

Unfortunately, the innate goodness of fruits and vegetables does not last forever. Fruits and vegetables begin to degrade from the moment they are picked and they continue to degrade in transit, in the store, and in your kitchen. If fresh fruits aren't available, canned and frozen foods are two alternatives.

Although fresh may be best, frozen is a very close second. Frozen fruits and vegetables sometimes have more vitamins and nutrients than the fresh variety because many are frozen soon after being picked, which helps to preserve the nutrients, although some nutrients may be lost in the freezing and thawing process.

Canning allows people to cheaply and conveniently enjoy foods that may have perished in less than a week for approximately two years. On the downside, canned food is cooked, preserved with salt and chemicals, and some nutrients are destroyed in the canning process.

Food supplies you with the energy and nutrients to live life. Although some foods give an immediate negative effect, there are some foods that go on years silently wreaking havoc on the inside of your body. Some people have a poor opinion of eating healthy, but it doesn't have to be so bad. You really don't have to miss out on anything. Too many factors like cravings, cost, and convenience often beat out nutrition and win a spot on the dinner table; however, nutrition must be a priority. A low-nutrient, high-calorie diet is a significant contributor to obesity. Not all food has the ability to fulfill nutritional requirements. Excess weight is not always about too much food, but it is about what you eat and how it affects your body. You only get one body; you have to take care of it so that it will take care of you. Let your desire to improve your health take over and tell your belly who's in charge of dinner. Good nutrition is a "thank you" to your body for all it does.

Salad

Eating salads is a great way to get the nutrients your body needs. However, you will not improve your health by eating any old salad. Salads come complete with landmines. If you don't want to do more harm than good then you have to take precautions. Yes, you can actually gain weight by eating salads.

First of all, the greener the better when it comes to lettuce. Dark green lettuces are low in calories, high in nutrients, and high in water. Iceberg lettuce, although highly popular in the US, is not very nutritious, but it is a good source of water.

Salad dressing can pack a load of calories and minimize the benefits of eating salad. Even low and reduced fat salad dressing may contain excess sugar to improve the taste lost from removing the fat. Vinaigrettes are good choices for dressings; they are made by mixing mono- and polyunsaturated oils, a variety of flavorful vinegars, and spices. Although unsaturated oils provide some benefits, use them sparingly. Oils are 100% fat and can ruin a good diet. To give you an idea exactly how fattening olive oil is, while a pound of butter has 3,200 calories, a pound of olive oil has 4,020 calories. Yikes!

A smorgasbord of toppings can liven up salads, but don't go overboard; more isn't always better. Cheese is a great addition to salads; however, many cheeses are high in saturated fat and not quite so healthy, so try to make a little cheese go a long way with strong cheeses like asiago and parmesan. Hard bread, also known as croutons, is a favorite salad topper. Go lightly or not at all with croutons. Depending on the crouton, it could be made from refined flour and trans-fat, which will add excess calories to your salad. Two or three ounces of an assortment of different proteins can be a welcome addition to salads. Some proteins that are frequently paired with salads include beef, chicken, shrimp, and tuna. Adding a protein can satisfy hunger longer and enhance the salad. Think about additions carefully to create a nutritious and delicious salad.

Although there is an investment of time and energy in preparing salads, the great news is that some lettuces like romaine can last up to 7 days when properly cleaned, packaged, and refrigerated. By pre-packing your salads you can have a meal ready in minutes.

Cooking vs. Raw

To reap all of the rewards innate in fruits and vegetables it may be necessary to eat them raw or lightly steamed. In addition, fresh uncooked fruits and vegetables provide the richest source of vitamins. Applying heat to food creates an endothermic chemical reaction, which alters the composition of food. Cooking often reduces and even destroys nutrients. Vitamins are delicate and easily destroyed with exposure to common elements like air, fats, heat, and water from food. Cooking some foods can result in the loss of 97% of water-soluble vitamins (B and C) and 40% of fat-soluble vitamins (A, D, E, and K), and may significantly reduce many other nutrients. Studies show that cooking may reduce the protein content of meat by 50%.

Diets high in raw foods are associated with weight loss and decreased blood pressure. In the past, those who focused entirely on a cooked diet without getting the proper allotment of fruits and vegetables suffered dismal fates by succumbing to scurvy and beriberi, diseases easily prevented by the nutrients within fruits. Studies show that raw foods provide the most protection against colon-related diseases. Additional studies show that people who eat raw fruits and vegetables are less likely to develop cancer than those people who primarily eat cooked food. Many researchers attribute autoimmune and degenerative diseases to not eating enough fruits and vegetables that heal and nourish the body.

It is extremely important to remove any chemicals, dirt, pesticides, or residue that may linger on fruits and vegetables. Rinsing with water is good, but cleansing in a sink with a tablespoon of salt and lemon is even better. If lemon isn't available, vinegar is a good alternative. Soak vegetables in a gallon of water with a tablespoon of vinegar. A boiling bath is also a good way to cleanse your vegetables. Quickly dunk fruits and vegetables into a vat of boiling water for a couple seconds.

Cooking food may produce a significant amount of harmful substances that may cause significant health complications. Studies have shown that heating fat causes significant chemical and physical changes. Heated fats promote cellular damage within the hearts, kidneys, and livers of lab animals. Using high temperatures to cook starch-rich foods forms acrylamide, which is a human carcinogen. Acrylamides are found in many foods such as baked potatoes, biscuits, breads, breakfast cereals, French fries, snack chips, and taco shells.

Advanced glycoxidation end products (AGEs) are harmful by-products of cooked foods. When cooking foods, the glucose binds to the protein. Studies show that 10% of AGEs are absorbed by the body and have a negative effect on the lens of the eyes and the heart muscle, which may cause a reduction in elasticity and stiffening of the tissue. The impact of AGEs has been found to be irreversible and may promote further damage in other protein bonds. AGEs are a common factor in food and responsible for the browning color of meats and toasts. Accumulated AGEs may cause brown spots on the skin.

Recent studies show that meats cooked at high temperatures and long durations generate mutagens and carcinogens in foods such as heterocyclic amines (HCAs), and polycyclic aromatic hydrocarbons (PAHs). Heterocyclic amines are a group of carcinogens produced from frying and grilling meat at high temperatures. Researchers believe there is a link between HCAs and colorectal cancer and other colon-related diseases.

PAHs are a group of chemicals formed from burning a series of substances like coal, exhaust, fire, food, fuel, tobacco, or volcanoes. PAHs may contaminate the air, soil, water, and a variety of foods to cause complications within the body. PAHs are known carcinogens (cancer causing agents), mutagens (agents that mutate genetic material), and teratogens (agents the damage embryos and fetuses).

While cooking some foods may reduce nutrients and create horrid by-products; it is beneficial to others. Tougher plant products like carrots, sweet potatoes, and tomatoes can withstand the heat and their nutrients are not destroyed. Cooking helps release the nutrients embodied in tomatoes and beans that are not readily available without cooking. Some foods like beans are less nutritious when raw; they contain enzymes that prevent protein digestion that are nonexistent after cooking. In addition, cooking makes some otherwise deadly foods safe by killing unsafe bacteria present on food.

Most minerals are not affected by heat, so don't worry about calcium, chromium, copper, phosphorus, magnesium, iron, zinc, iodine, selenium, manganese, or sodium. The mineral to look out for is potassium; it may migrate from the food to the broth.

Organic

Foods and animals grown with less or no harsh chemicals and that have not been irradiated or bio-engineered earn an organic food label. Fertilizers, pesticides, and herbicides try to enhance produce, yet often use harsh chemicals to get the job done. Governmental agencies condone the use of a smorgasbord of chemicals to enhance crops by rationalizing that it's not really that *much* poison, it's just a little poison—it should be fine—or so we all hope. This is one of the many reasons to eat organic foods. The following fruits and vegetables are regularly contaminated with herbicides and pesticides:

Apples	Cherries	Peaches	Raspberries
Bell peppers	Grapes	Pears	Spinach
Celery	Nectarines	Potatoes	Strawberries

While organic foods are grown with fewer or no chemicals, studies from the England and Food Standard Agency show that there is no significant nutritional difference between organic and nonorganic foods; however, over the last 100 years we have learned that chemicals have latent negative effects on the human body and may be potentially lethal. The avoidance of chemicals is particularly important to children, especially during their formative years.

Of course, like everything, organic foods have their problems as well. Without the pesticides, there may be icky bugs crawling on the food; bugs get hungry too. Some studies report that Americans actually consume a pound or two of insects per year ground up in foods like jams, peanut butters, and sauces. But on the bright side, insects are low in fat and cholesterol, are nutritious, and frequently eaten in Asia.

"An average of two rodent hairs per one hundred grams of peanut butter is allowed."
— No. 20. FDA GOVERNMENT GUIDELINES

Many grocery stores are beginning to carry a larger variety of organic foods. If you cannot find certain organic items, search the health food stores and online. Buying organic foods can be expensive, they may cost two to three times the amount of nonorganic foods, but health food stores may provide cheaper prices than traditional grocery stores on some organic foods.

Fiber

If you are being treated for a medical condition, consult with your doctor before increasing your daily fiber.

Fiber is the edible, yet indigestible parts of plants that facilitates digestion. Unlike protein, which is found in animals and plant products, fiber is only found in plant products. Fiber, like complex carbohydrates, is made of multiple units of sugar; however, the units cannot be broken down by human digestive enzymes and is not a source of calories, energy, or nutrition. High-fiber foods have more bulk than low-fiber foods and promote feelings of fullness. Fiber moves through the body slowly, which promotes satiety, reduces overeating, and assists in regulating blood sugar.

Partial fermentation of the fiber occurs in the colon when bacteria break down fiber to produce acids and gases, which nourish the lining of the colon. The acids and gases from fermentation soften and enlarge the stool, which may cause bloating for some people while the rest are expelled. When adding fiber to your diet it is important to drink more water. Fiber absorbs large amounts of water in the bowels and this makes stools softer and easier to pass. Without sufficient water, there may be a stall in the pipes. To avoid bloating, constipation, cramping, or gas, slowly add fiber to your diet over a couple of weeks.

Fiber is not easily destroyed. Unlike delicate vitamins, fiber can withstand canning, cooking, drying, and freezing; however, the milling and refining process leaves many fiber-rich products virtually fiber-less, especially flour.

The American diet is severely deficient in fiber, with an average consumption of only 12–18 grams per day. The United States National Academy of Sciences, Institute of Medicine, and the ADA recommend 20–35 grams of fiber per day. Many experts believe low fiber consumption is a significant contributor to the obesity crisis and health complications.

Fiber is a great food to incorporate into daily meals when trying to lose weight because it maintains stable sugar levels and satisfies hunger while not adding too many calories. Fiber delays the absorption of glucose and thereby alleviates the workload of the pancreas. Fiber helps transport cholesterol and bile out of the body. Without fiber, cholesterol and bile may be reabsorbed by the body. While adding fiber to your diet, carefully review food labels to determine the fiber content. Some high-fiber foods like breakfast cereals and snacks are also high in sugar and salt.

Fiber is an important part of the diet; however, dietary needs change as you age.

Daily Fiber Requirement

	Women < 51	Men < 51	Women > 51	Men > 51
Grams of Fiber	25	38	21	30

Fiber helps relieve constipation and hemorrhoids, manage weight, and prevent certain diseases such as cancer, diabetes, diverticular disease, gallstones, heart disease, and kidney stones. Fiber protects against many ailments like appendicitis, candida, colitis, diabetes, gallstones, heart disease, high blood pressure, high cholesterol, and irritable bowel syndrome. Without enough fiber, you may become susceptible to colon-related diseases including, but not limited to: colon cancer, diverticulosis, and hemorrhoids

Constipation is the most significant gastrointestinal issue in the US. Constipation sufferers make over two million trips to the doctor and spend close to a billion dollars in over-the-counter medications to relieve their clogged pipes, when a healthy diet filled with fiber is the best cure. If increasing fiber does not alleviate constipation, there may be other complications and consulting with a doctor may help.

Reducing dairy, meats, and refined and processed carbohydrates can significantly improve your gastrointestinal health. Now don't get turned off by the word reduce, it's not the word eliminate, you can eat them again. Fiber-less products may include juice, pasta, pizza crusts, and white breads. Fruits and vegetables are refined for their juice, while their fiber content is discarded. *Reducing* dairy, meat, and refined and processed carbohydrates will help you make room for fiber. Fiber provides so many benefits you may want to call it your BFF—Best Friend Fiber.

Take this pill or drink this concoction to get the same benefits of fiber. Yeah right! It's just not that easy to get the real thing into synthetic replacements. Supplements provide only a very limited amount of fiber. There are hundreds of different substances that make up fiber and the benefits are created through a series of complex biochemical and physiological reactions within the body. Through scientific means, a couple of the actions can be replicated; however, they do not emulate the compound effects of fiber; there is no substitute for the real thing.

Research studies show that high-fiber diets have numerous health benefits; however, to reap bountiful benefits both soluble and insoluble fiber should be consumed. Insoluble fiber is mainly composed of the cell walls of plants, which cannot be dissolved in water and is a good laxative. Soluble fiber is made up of carbohydrates that contain three or more molecules of simple carbohydrates known as polysaccharides, which dissolve in water. Soluble fiber absorbs water to form a gelatinous substance that passes through the body.

Insoluble fibers

+ Lignans
+ Flax seed
+ Potato skins
+ Nuts and seeds
+ Whole grain foods
+ Wheat and corn bran
+ Skins of some fruits, including tomatoes
+ Vegetables such as cauliflower, celery, green beans, nopal, and zucchini (courgette)

Soluble fibers

+ Fruits (some)
+ Psyllium seed husk
+ Barley, chia, oats, and rye
+ Legumes (peas, soybeans, and other beans)
+ Vegetables (broccoli, carrots, and Jerusalem artichokes)
+ Root vegetables like potatoes, onions, and sweet potatoes (skins of these vegetables are sources of insoluble fiber)

Psyllium fiber is a good source of unsweetened and unflavored fiber that can be mixed with liquid. Psyllium fiber can be purchased at most health food stores.

Most low-fiber foods have a higher-fiber alternative:

If you like these low-fiber foods	Try these high-fiber foods
Sweetened cereal	Shredded wheat, puffed wheat
White bread	Whole-grain bread
Snack cakes	Whole-grain muffins
Snack crackers	Wheat crackers
Fruit juice	Fresh or frozen fruit
Cakes, biscuits, sweets	Dried fruit, nuts, raw carrots, oatmeal
Puddings	Blended fruits
Jam	Nut butters (cashew, almond, etc.)

The benefits of unrefined natural fiber include, but are not limited to:

+ Facilitates digestion
+ Promotes regularity
+ Regulates blood sugar
+ Regulate intestinal pH
+ Improve immune functions
+ Improves glucose absorption

+ Reduces risk of heart disease
+ Improves gastrointestinal health
+ Stimulates intestinal fermentation
+ Reduces total and LDL cholesterol
+ Alleviates and helps prevent constipation
+ Reduces the risk of developing some cancers
+ Reduces inflammation and adhesion of irritants
+ Improves glucose tolerance and insulin sensitivity
+ Improves barrier protection of the colonic mucosal layer
+ May reduce onset risk or symptoms of metabolic syndrome and diabetes
+ Attracts water to form gel to trap carbohydrates and slow the absorption of glucose
+ Adds bulk to your diet, making you feel full faster and helps with weight management
+ Lowers colonic pH which protects the lining from the formation of colonic polyps and increases absorption of dietary minerals

Although fiber is an important part of the diet, some studies show consuming too much fiber can impede the absorption of many amino acids, minerals, nutrients, and vitamins needed by the body. Fiber is very absorptive; it has the ability to remove toxins, but it also has the ability to absorb medications as well; therefore, plan your meals and medications appropriately or you may miss your dose. More than 45 grams of fiber per day may cause complications; remember, moderation is key with everything.

Whole Grains

Fruits and vegetables are not the only source of fiber; whole grains are also a good option. Whole grains are an important part of the diet, yet more than 80% of Americans eat less than one serving per day.

Incorporating whole grains can be as easy as starting the day with a bowl of whole grain cereal. Select a cereal that has at least five grams or more; this should be easy considering some cereals contain up to 20 grams of fiber per serving. Look at the fiber content on the nutrition label to find the cereal right for you.

All whole grains are not beneficial. To reap the health benefits, it is important that whole grains have limited refining and processing. With limited processing, food maintains it original nutrients. Moreover, when food is refined, it is more easily absorbed in the body and quickly raises glucose levels, which may promote fat storage. However, unrefined carbohydrates are absorbed slowly and may satisfy hunger longer.

Another way to add whole grains to your diet is to replace flour, rice, and potatoes with bulgur, wheat berries, and other whole grains. Experiment with replacing some of your meals with whole grain alternatives.

The flour that most of us have come to love is composed of whole grains. The innermost layer of a whole grain is known as the endosperm. The two outermost layers, the bran, a.k.a. outer shell with all of its good stuff like fiber and B vitamins, and the germ, with the phytochemicals, have been removed. Vigilance is necessary when selecting good whole wheat options. Many advertisers promote whole wheat when it is not a major component of the product. When buying whole grain products, review the list of ingredients to ensure that the main ingredients include whole wheat, whole oats, whole rye, but not enriched flour or similar ingredients. Wheat flour is not the same as whole wheat. Even if a label claims the product is made with whole wheat, it doesn't mean it is 100% whole wheat. Labels can be tricky. Turn that package over and get some more information.

Label	Possible Meaning
Made with whole grains	Only has a to have a speck
100% whole wheat	Could mean it has a speck of 100% whole wheat
Multigrain	Could be refined grains
Whole grain	May be blended with refined, processed, or enriched products
Blends	Not 100% whole grains
Good source	Eight grams of whole grams per serving
Excellent source	16 grams of whole grains per serving
Supports health	Any food can claim this; however, a stronger claim is "May reduce the risk."

Gluten

Gluten is a special protein mainly found in barley, rye, and wheat; it may also be in lip balms, medicines, and vitamins. Gluten is only bad for your health if you can't properly digest it like individuals with gluten allergies, gluten intolerance, or celiac disease. There are many wheat alternatives that do not have gluten including amaranth, buckwheat, corn, millet, oats, quinoa, soybeans, sunflower seeds, teff, and wild rice.

Gluten sensitivity may promote an allergic reaction that causes the immune system to damage the tiny, finger-like protrusions lining the small intestine, known as villi. Villi absorb nutrients through the walls of the small intestine into the bloodstream. Without nutrient absorption from healthy villi, malnutrition may develop, despite adequate nourishment. Malnutrition can lead to anemia, cancer, liver disease, miscarriage, and osteoporosis.

Celiac disease is an autoimmune disease of the small intestine that is aggravated by gluten and similar products, which results in gastro-intestinal problems. Although celiac disease was once thought to be a rare childhood syndrome, it is now known to be a common genetic disorder. More than two million people in the US suffer from celiac disease, or about one in 133 people. Many people have ranges of gluten sensitivity without having celiac disease. Celiac disease may develop after a pregnancy, severe emotional stress, surgery, or viral infection. Only a doctor or geneticist can properly diagnosis celiac disease.

Celiac disease promotes the development of other diseases that may damage the body's healthy cells and tissues including:

+ Type I diabetes
+ Rheumatoid arthritis
+ Autoimmune disease
+ Addison's disease, the glands that produce critical hormones are damaged
+ Sjögren's syndrome, the glands that produce tears and saliva are destroyed

The treatment for gluten-related problems is a gluten-free diet. Avoiding gluten makes eating more challenging. Although manufacturers attempt to remove gluten, 100% of gluten cannot be removed; however, products may be labeled "gluten-free" with limited amounts of gluten present. Gluten sensitive individuals may suffer after consuming foods that are improperly labeled gluten free or have been grown or processed near gluten. If you have a wheat allergy it is time to get perceptive—read all labels to determine the content. When dining out, inform your waiter you have a wheat allergy. Eat more fruits and vegetables to avoid gluten. When you have your own snacks, you aren't at the mercy of foods that may be contaminated with gluten.

Nuts

Most nuts, minus chestnuts, are a good source of fiber, minerals, protein, and vitamins. Nuts like chestnuts, pecans, and walnuts have high amounts of antioxidants. Some nuts like almonds also help regulate blood sugar. Researchers from the Nurses' Health Study found that there may be a 30% reduction in heart disease by substituting nuts for refined carbohydrates.

All nuts have large quantities of beneficial mono- and polyunsaturated fats. Although nuts contain healthy oils, they are oils nonetheless that contain many calories and can be fattening, despite beneficial factors. Nuts may quickly become rancid; therefore, it is best to eat nuts quickly after buying or shelling them, or store them in a refrigerator where they may last from 6 to 12 months. Old nuts may not present any tell-tale signs like bad smell or taste; but they may become rancid and have greater quantities of body-damaging free radicals.

Nuts come in a variety of delicious textures, spices, and versatile options such as à la carte, sprinkled over salads and vegetables, roasted in the oven, buttered, roasted, sliced, dipped, spiced, dusted, coated, and blended with drinks, fruits, salads, rices, whole grain breads, and yogurts.

As you can imagine, not all of enhancements to nuts are healthy. Watch out for the nuts covered with chocolate, salt, and sugar, which may add more calories. Nut butter is a good source of protein; however, it generally contains a significant amount of calories, fat, and sugar. Don't let the healthiness or small size fool you; a single serving of six to ten nuts can pack a heap of protein and calories. Roasting nuts for 10–15 minutes at 160–175 degrees may enhance the flavor of nuts, reduce the rancidness, and ease digestion. Although the heat may reduce some of the antioxidants in the nuts, it will not deplete them. In addition, almonds contain oxalates, natural substances found in many animals and plants; in high amounts they may crystallize and aggravate kidney or gallbladder problems and may interfere with calcium absorption.

Beans

Unlike meats, beans provide much more like: calcium, fiber, folate, minerals, potassium, protein, and vitamins. In addition to being an inexpensive source of protein, beans are virtually fat free. Beans are very versatile and can be prepared in a myriad of ways like casseroles, chili, desserts, dips, salads, spreads, soups, and stews.

Beans may promote indigestion and flatulence; however, these negative side effects may be reduced or eliminated by taking a few precautions:

+ Choose the right bean
  ◇ Easy to digest beans can be enjoyed regularly: aduki, lentils, mung, and peas
  ◇ Harder to digest beans can be enjoyed occasionally: black-eyed peas, garbanzo, kidney, lima, navy, and pinto
  ◇ Difficult to digest beans: soybeans and black soybeans; the processed versions are easier to digest, which include: miso, soybean sprouts, soy milk, soy sauce, tempeh, and tofu.
+ Season with fennel or cumin
+ Chew your beans thoroughly
+ Reduce the quantity of beans that you eat
+ Soak beans overnight or at least 12 hours
+ Cook with some seaweed like kombu or kelp

Types of Beans

adzuki	navy beans	brown lentils
split peas	pinto beans	kidney beans
red lentils	white beans	haricot beans
red beans	green lentils	green beans
soybeans	black beans	garbanzo beans
lima beans	butter beans	yellow split peas
fava beans	broad beans	great northern bean
black-eyed peas	mung beans	

Soy

Soybeans have been a staple of some Asian countries for thousands of years. Soybeans are low in saturated fat and a good source of minerals, omega-3 fatty acids, protein, and vitamins. Soybeans are quite versatile creating butters, flours, and oils. Tofu and roasted soybeans make tasty treats.

There are many health benefits associated with eating soybeans including reducing cholesterol, heart disease, menopause-related issues; preserving mental faculties; and protecting against some forms of cancer. Soybeans contain phytoestrogens, which are plant estrogens, isoflavones, and lignans. Soy has received some acclaim for its ability to relieve menopausal symptoms. Phytoestrogens may mimic estrogen or block the effects of estrogen, which may provide protection against breast cancer.

While there are benefits to eating soy, there are also studies that show consuming large amounts of soy may be detrimental to one's health by promoting certain cancers. Soy can also negatively affect the thyroid and may cause hypothyroidism, which may hinder weight loss efforts. Moreover, studies show years of high soy consumption may lead to an increased risk of dementia. Therefore, as with almost everything, moderation is key.

Sea Plants

Seaweed comes in a variety of colors and generally contains 10 to 20 times more vitamins and nutrients than land plants. Seaweed alkalizes the blood, cleanses and detoxifies the body, reduces fats and cholesterol, and reduces solid masses within the body like glands, goiters, lumps, and swollen areas. Nutrient rich seaweed includes, but is not limited to: agar-agar, corsican, dulse, hijiki, Irish moss, kelp, kombu, nori, and wakame.

To prepare seaweed, soak it in water to reduce the salt content and facilitate digestion. Seaweed can be added to a variety of foods like casseroles, dressings, greens, rice rolls, sandwiches, soups, and stir fry; but there is no limit on how you can prepare it. Experiment with adding seaweed to different dishes to increase the nutritional value of any meal. Although you may be eager to reap the benefits of seaweed, gradually add it to your diet to give your body time to adjust to the new addition.

Conclusion

Plant products provide a plethora of options to feed, nourish, and heal the body; however, good decisions must be made. Plant products are not all good. To improve health, it is important to reduce or eliminate refined and processed plant products, while filling up on natural, unrefined plant products.

Animal Products 6

Red Meat

Millions of people enjoy the taste, texture, and the satiation of meat. Years ago in many countries, meat was considered a rarity; mainly enjoyed by the elite while most people could only afford to consume it on the rare occasion. Meat eating has been associated with having wealth while eating plant products is associated with being poor. These connotations still exist in some forms today. However, stereotypes and other erroneous values should not be the driving force behind any diet.

Many critics believe that if wild animals like lions and tigers can live relatively well on no carbs and meat, then why can't we? Well, for one, *most* of us aren't wild animals. A lion or tiger's life span averages 10–16 years in the wild, and up to 26 in captivity. Lions and tigers are fierce, ferocious hunters designed to catch their nimble and fleeting prey and then pierce them with their razor-sharp canine teeth. These carnivores have a significant amount of hydrochloric acid present in their stomach to help digest meat, accompanied by a short intestinal tract to dispel it with ease; otherwise, if they had a long intestinal tract like we have, meat would be sitting there, rotting, decaying, and possibly promoting a series of unsavory conditions.

Many people often attempt to increase their physical prowess through increased meat consumption. Those who wantonly enjoy meat may suffer more cancer, diabetes, and heart disease. Meat is often referred to as the "higher quality" protein; however, plants are just as capable as meat at helping anyone reach the pinnacle of physical potential, while helping to prevent cancer, obesity, and other illnesses.

Some health gurus recommend limiting meat. Most Americans consume more meat than required by the body. The body obtains protein from multiple sources such as itself, carbohydrates, and meat. Most standard servings provide more meat than necessary. The 16 ounce steak at your favorite restaurant is way too much. Only four ounces is needed per serving for men and only three ounces for ladies.

You don't have to be a vegetarian to reach your weight goals; a moderate reduction in the amount of meat you consume can improve your health and help you lose weight. Studies show that meat eaters gain significantly more weight than vegetarians and are more likely to overeat. Some research studies conclude that many vegetarians eat more than meat eaters, yet are slimmer and healthier. Additional studies show that those who partake in a diet low in meat and high in fruits and vegetables were less fatigued, exercised more voluntarily, and had better weight management. As an added bonus, consuming less meat provides ecological benefits by reducing the demand for land and water, while reducing pollution.

Researchers have concluded that cultures that consume greater amounts of meat are at a higher risk for developing tumors in the large bowel, 10% of which will develop into a malignancy. A diet rich in meats and refined foods, while low in fruits and vegetables, also promotes the growth of uterine fibroids.

The Insulin-like Growth Factor I (IGF-1) is a hormone made by the body that under unhealthy conditions has the ability to promote cancer growth while impeding the removal of old cells. Unfortunately, eating meat increases the presence of IGF-1.

Unlike plant products, meats increase the acidity of the body. The body strives to maintain a slightly alkaline pH of 7.35 pH level; to do so the body may leach calcium from the bones, which causes a series of problems including breaks, fractures, and osteoporosis. This occurrence is further validated by research data that shows that countries with less meat consumption also have fewer bone-related breaks. Not to mention, the excess calcium is excreted in urine, which may promote the development of kidney stones.

Eating a diet high in meat affects hormone levels; however, plant products do not pose the same risk. Hormone levels are especially important to women during menopause. During menopause the hormone levels of women drop significantly; however, the drop is not as significant for women who reduce meat consumption and eat more fruits and vegetables. Women who experience extreme changes in hormone levels endure more uncomfortable conditions that lead them to search for pharmaceutical cures. Hormone replacement therapy (HRT) is one the cures that women utilize to treat the symptoms of menopause; however this cure has consequences. The Women's Health Initiative (WHI) and the Heart and Estrogen/Progestin Replacement Study (HERS) conclude that using hormone replacement therapy may increase the risk of contracting breast cancer by 25 to 30%. To naturally reduce negative symptoms associated with menopause it is important to consume a diet low in fat and meat and increase plant products.

Researchers have also found that eating red meat increases estrogen levels. This is alarming because there is a significant correlation with high estrogen levels and the development of breast cancer. Women who eat large amounts of meat may be at greater risk for contracting breast cancer. Some researchers believe that high dietary fat also increases estrogen levels, and thereby makes women more susceptible to breast cancer. This relationship is strengthened by the low occurrences of breast cancers in countries that have low dietary fat intake.

Moooo!

Most dairy farmers want as much bang for the buck as possible, so farm animals are given steroids and growth hormones to increase the quantity of milk production. Recombinant bovine somatropin is a genetically engineered growth hormone that stimulates the production of milk. Although many countries have banned the use of the hormone because of the increased risk of cancer, it is still approved for use in the US. The people who inadvertently drink milk laced with steroids and hormones do not go unaffected. Growth hormones and steroids promote weight gain, the early onset of puberty for children, and possibly other problems which have yet to be realized. Some of the growth hormones from cows are believed to promote the growth of cancer in humans.

As if steroids and drugs weren't hazardous enough, chemical pesticides are used directly on the skin of animals to protect them against a variety of fungi, insects, parasites, and rodents. Farm animals get another dose of chemical pesticides from eating food that has been treated with chemical pesticides. Meats designated as suitable for consumption can arrive to your dinner table with over 100 different pesticide residues.

Although pesticides are regularly used on plant products, studies show that meats contain 14 times more pesticides than dairy and five times more pesticides than fruits and vegetables. The pesticides and chemicals used on animals have been known to promote a series of problems such as: decreased metabolism, increased appetite, reduced ability to lose stored fat, and reduced desire to exercise. No wonder many European countries will not accept animal product importations from the US.

Free-range diets are optimal for cattle; however, they don't all receive this type of diet. Some animals are given unnatural and

unhealthy diets to fatten them quickly. Feedlots feed and house hundreds to thousands of livestock before slaughter. The feedlot system confines livestock and feeds them a grain-based diet or scraps of garbage left over from human meals like pastries, ice cream, and even meat. Cows can gain approximately 400 pounds in about three to six months. Although the feedlot system is economical, allowing farmers to earn profits while keeping consumer prices low, the system confines livestock to overcrowded, squalid quarters.

Improper diets and unsanitary conditions cause animals to develop a series of health problems like subacute acidosis and malnourishment that causes the animals to eat dirt, which increases the need for antibiotics to protect against bacteria, filth, and fecal matter. Cattle require almost half of the antibiotics consumed in the US each year, which promotes antibiotic resistance in humans.

Grain and garbage-fed livestock produce meat with lower nutritional values, more calories, more cholesterol, and more saturated fat while having less beta carotene, omega-3 fatty acids, and vitamins. Free-range grass-fed animals offer significant benefits which include, but are not limited to: leaner meat with as much as one third less fat, fewer calories, more beneficial omega-3 fatty acid, more vitamins, and more conjugated linoleic acid (CLA). CLA is a fatty acid found in the meat and whole dairy products of grazing animals. CLA is especially important to dieters because it limits the body's ability to store fat while improving the body's ability to develop muscle from fat. Studies also show that CLA also helps fight cancer.

You don't have to give up meat to be healthy. Meat provides vitamins and minerals that cannot be found in other sources. It is true that vitamin manufacturers attempt to replicate the vitamins and minerals in meat known to be beneficial; however, research shows us every day that there is always something new to be discovered.

If you are fond of meat, it is important to incorporate plant products into your diet to neutralize the acidifying effect of meats.

In addition, you can significantly reduce the fat content by selecting leaner cuts of meat. Lean cuts of meat generally have less saturated fat. Fat is white, so when you're cooking steak, cut off the fat to reduce the calories. If you're buying pink ground meat, watch out. Butchers grind red meat and white fat, to produce tasty, yet fattening, pink meat. Eating 12 ounces or less of lean meat per week may help improve your health.

Marbling is the white saturated fat intermingled between cuts of meat. Without marbling, meat may be dry and flavorless. When cooked, the marbled fat disperses through the meat creating, juicy tender meat. A fair amount of marbling does enhance the flavor and improve the texture; however, too much marbling not only will not provide any excess enhancements, but may also promote health complications.

Some cattle are bred and fed to ensure the development of marbled meat. Marbling is achieved by quickly fattening up cattle on a cereal and grain diet; however, optimally cattle should eat a free-range grass diet. As ruminants, cattle have digestive systems made to promote the digestion of grass, not grains like barley and corn. Not all cattle tolerate grains. Specific cattle are raised to produce marbled meat like Angus, Murray Grey, Shorthorns, and Wagyu type cattle; and dairy breeds such as the Jersey, Holstein-Friesian, and Braunvieh.

There is even a marbling hierarchy that awards the highest designation to the meats with the most marbling. From the highest to the lowest the designations are prime, choice, select, standard, commercial, utility, cutter, and canner. Red meat doesn't have to be the wicked culprit that it is made out to be. If you are trying to improve your health, it may be best to forgo the best cuts of meat. By picking a cut of meat with limited marbling can be both tasty and a good source of protein.

White meat is sometimes perceived as a healthier and less fattening meat alternative; however, studies have found that red meat is just as healthy as white meat, maybe even healthier because cooked chicken contain 15 times more heterocyclic amines, a carcinogen formed from heated animal protein. In addition, red meat can be just as healthy as chicken by selecting leaner cuts of meat. Chicken and turkey skin is a considerable source of fat; however, leaving it on while cooking may provide protection from the heat while enhancing the flavor of the food; but remember to take it off before eating.

Fish

Most fish does not contain a lot of fat. Fish is a good source of omega-3 fatty acids, especially for individuals with thickened arterial walls due to plaque buildup, also known as atherosclerosis. Life threatening clots called thrombi can form in the plaque. If a thrombus travels, it is then called an embolus. Generally, thrombi and emboli are the cause of heart attacks and strokes. One or two servings of fish like halibut, mackerel, salmon, sardines, and trout per week provide the omega-3 fatty acids needed to help reduce blood clots; however, more servings have not been found to reduce blood clots.

Fish can be packaged and prepared a number of different ways; of course, some are better for your health than others. Tuna and sardines packed in oil contain more calories than water based tuna, which is a better option. While fried fish may be appetizing, the oil packs excessive calories; baking, broiling, and grilling fish are better cooking styles. Properly seasoning fish can enhance the taste. A splash of fresh lemon, lime, or orange, with a dash of salt, pepper, and garlic powder can create a mouth-watering entrée that can please the finickiest eater.

Although fish offers benefits, it does come with some drawbacks. Fish oil may cause the vessels in the brain to bleed, causing a hemorrhagic stroke. Large fish like shark, swordfish, and blue and yellow fin tuna contain particularly high contaminant levels, which may cause cancer. Eating fish more than twice per week may impose increased health risks, especially for young children and pregnant women. The toxins found in fish can result in a series of health complications including, but not limited to cancers, fertility complications, neurological damage, and suppressed immunological response.

Fish also contains contaminants from pesticide residue, waste products, and environmental pollutants such as BHC, chlordane, DDT, mercury, and PCB. Polychlorinated Biphenyls (PCBs) are known carcinogens. Although the manufacture of PCBs was banned in the US in 1979, machinery with PCBs was allowed to continue operating. PCBs have low solubility and are found in water, but are not absorbed into water because they are lipophilic (fat soluble) and accumulate heavily in aquatic organisms. PCBs not only accumulate in fish, but in red meat and dairy products. Dredging, evaporation, and flooding allow PCBs to be found throughout the earth in the air, animal tissue, sediment, soil, and water.

When eating fish carefully consider the type, origin, and possible contaminants.

Least Mercury			
Anchovies	Haddock (Atlantic)	Pollock	Squid (Calamari)
Butterfish	Hake	Salmon (Canned)*	Tilapia
Catfish	Herring	Salmon (Fresh)*	Trout (Freshwater)
Clam	Mackerel (N. Atlantic, Chub)	Sardine	Whitefish
Crab (Domestic)	Mullet	Scallop	Whiting
Crawfish	Oyster	Shad (American)	
Croaker (Atlantic)	Perch (Ocean)	Shrimp	
Flounder	Plaice	Sole (Pacific)	

*contains PCBs

Moderate Mercury		
Bass (Striped, Black)	Jacksmelt	Silverside

Carp	Lobster	Skate
Cod (Alaskan)	Mahi Mahi	Snapper
Croaker (White Pacific)	Monkfish	Tuna (Canned chunk light)
Halibut (Atlantic)	Perch (Freshwater)	Tuna (Skipjack)
Halibut (Pacific)	Sablefish	Weakfish (Sea Trout)

High Mercury		
Bluefish	Mackerel (Spanish, Gulf)	Tuna (Canned Albacore)
Grouper	Sea Bass (Chilean)	Tuna (Yellowfin)

Highest Mercury		
Mackerel (King)	Shark	Tuna (Bigeye, Ahi)
Marlin	Swordfish	
Orange Roughy	Tilefish	

Conclusion

While it is not necessary for you to abandon meat, it is prudent to carefully consider multiple factors before eating meat like the quantity and quality of the meat consumed. Good choices may significantly reduce your risk for several diseases, and thereby improve your health.

There is a way for you to have your meat and eat it too. Meat is not all bad. There are many societies of people who experience longevity and good health while enjoying the carnal fruit. Several factors can reduce the negative effects associated with meat, such as the portion size of meat, the type of meat being consumed, and the addition of plant products to your diet. Before completely abstaining from meat, consider all of the ways that you can make eating meat a healthier option for you.

Inside Plants and Meats 7

Casein

Casein is the main protein found in dairy products and is also used in a variety of foods and medicines because of its binding properties. Cheese typically has the highest amount of casein. Casein has been known to cause allergic reactions. Some people look for lactose free foods to avoid casein; however, even soy and lactose-free foods may still contain it.

There are some scientists who believe that casein significantly increases the risk of developing cancer. Under experimental conditions casein has been found to increase atherosclerotic plaque, cancer growth, and cholesterol levels. Research scientists observed the cancer levels of rats increase when fed diets high in casein and decrease when fed diets low in casein. In addition, research has shown that individuals with autism are especially sensitive to casein because when digested it has a morphine or opiate-like effect.

Fat

In the last few decades, people have eaten less and less fat, while eating more carbohydrates like rice, pasta, and flour to replace the alleged bad bad fat, but as we have seen, replacing the fat in foods with refined carbohydrates has not done much for everyone's waistline.

For years the public has been warned against the evils of oils and fats, yet this information does not provide the complete picture. Although lowering fat intake is important, it is not sufficient to lose weight and provide significant improvements to your health.

Although fat is generally thought of as yucky, useless, and the source to most of our dietary woes, it has many important functions within the body. Although you can't eat all you want, fat is a good and necessary part of the diet. Fat is located throughout the body. The brain is approximately 60% fat and the outer membranes of many internal structures are composed of fat. The body uses fat to insulate membranes, and when it does not find it, the body searches for replacements, which may be unsuitable. It is no wonder why the body craves and needs fat daily to operate optimally.

Total fat is not as important as type of fat. Some fats are better than others. Good (unsaturated) fats reduce the body's inflammatory response while bad fats (saturated) increase the body's inflammatory response. It is important to consume adequate amounts of fat to aid essential processes and to allow the body to release stored fat. Fat also helps absorb and use fat soluble vitamins that help the immune system, reproductive organs, skin, and vision.

A multi-country study of fat intake found that women who consumed low amounts of fat were more likely to be obese. Reducing saturated fats while increasing unsaturated fats like olives, nuts, and seeds, can provide many benefits like:

+ Reduce risk for blood clots
+ Lower LDL (bad cholesterol)
+ Reduce the risk of arrhythmia
+ Prevent increases in triglycerides (fat in the blood)

In general, the French consume lots of fatty foods, yet do not suffer the same obesity rates found in the US. Studies reveal that while French people do indulge in fatty foods, they do not consume nearly as much as Americans. On average, Americans consume 35–40% of total calories from fat. It is not necessary for you to abstain from the foods that you love, but it is necessary to reduce the quantity, especially if they are not good for your health.

Oils are 100% liquid fat; therefore, even healthy oils should be used sparingly. Some oils spoil quickly, so refrigeration is important. Although refrigerated oils may thicken and cloud, they quickly return to their original condition at room temperature. When cooking, it's good to apply oils last to ensure the oil is not damaged.

You don't have to search hard to get fat into your diet; it's in everything tasty like diary, meat, oils, poultry, and processed foods. All fats are not created equally. Let's review the good (unsaturated), the bad (saturated), and the ugly (trans) fats.

Although there are no safe amounts of saturated fat, ideally, diets should contain miniscule amounts of saturated fats. Saturated fats are a main culprit for causing heart disease and cancers. Health experts recommend consuming less than 10% of the daily calories from saturated fats and less than four grams of saturated fat per serving. Dairy, meat, and oil are the main sources of saturated fat. Saturated fat is solid at room temperature. Oils high in saturated fat include: coconut 91%, lard 43%, and palm 51%, while butter contains 68%.

Unsaturated fats include monounsaturated and polyunsaturated fats. Used in place of saturated fats, monounsaturated, and even poly-unsaturated fats are beneficial. Unsaturated fats improve cholesterol levels, and thereby reduce the risk for heart disease. Monounsaturated fats are liquid at room temperature. Oils with high monounsaturated content include canola, olive, and peanut. Monounsaturated oils are also found in a variety of plant products like avocados and nuts. Although better than saturated fat, unsaturated fats are still oils and are therefore not good in copious amounts.

Omega-9, including oleic and stearic acid, is a monounsaturated non-essential fatty acid that the body can produce from unsaturated fats within the body. Omega-9 is able to: lower cholesterol, reduce atherosclerosis, reduce insulin resistance, improve immune function, and help protect against certain cancers. Omega-9 can be found in the following foods:

Avocados	Cashews	Olives and olive oil
Almonds	Hazelnuts	Peanuts
Brazil nuts	Macadamia nuts	Sesame seeds

Not as good as monounsaturated fat, but not as bad as saturated fats; polyunsaturated fats include a variety of oils including corn, safflower, soybean, and sunflower. Polyunsaturated fats are liquid at room temperature and chilled.

There are multiple processes used to extract oil from seeds; however, methods that utilize chemicals and heat extraction may damage the oil. Expeller and cold pressed oils have not been refined and offer more benefits than processed oils. Extra virgin denotes the oil has not been adulterated through refining and processing, and therefore is a better quality and more pure oil.

Mono- and polyunsaturated vegetable oils have a short shelf life and may grow rancid rapidly; however, adding hydrogen molecules stabilizes them, extends their shelf life, and increases their flash point to cook at higher temperatures. Hydrogenating mono- and polyunsaturated oils vilifies them, making them into partially hydrogenated oil, less like good unsaturated oils and more like bad saturated oil and otherwise known as trans-fat.

Although trans-fat is not found in nature, it is found regularly in the American diet. The Harvard Nurses' Study regards trans-fat as more than twice as detrimental to health versus saturated fat because it promotes a series of negative health complications including inflammation, insulin resistance, and leptin resistance. Trans and saturated fats both raise the level of LDL and triglycerides in the blood, which ignites inflammation, promotes damage to arteries, and may eventually cause heart disease.

Trans-fat is an artificial creation that can pretty easily be eliminated from your diet. While there are no safe amounts of trans-fat, most nutritional experts recommend less than two grams per day; however, most foods with trans-fat tend to have significantly more than recommended. Fried chicken has 10 grams while imitation cheese has eight grams. Traditional margarine is a trans-fat and is worse for your health than butter, a saturated fat. Some of the new margarines have revised their contents to remove the unhealthy trans-fat. Nonetheless, it is important to review the label to ensure the contents do not contain trans-fat.

Fatty Acids

Although the American diet has plenty of fat, the right kind of fat is eaten in infinitesimal amounts or not at all. Dietary research studies have shown that good fats are essential to maintaining optimal health. Polyunsaturated fats known as EFAs (essential fatty acids) are required for cells to develop and function, as well as to protect and guard against chronic diseases. It is estimated as much as 80% of American diets are deficient in essential fatty acids. Bodies with insufficient amounts of EFAs may be more likely to develop cancer, cardiovascular disease, depression, diabetes, eczema, fatigue, joint pain, mental complications, and weak hair and nails.

Although the body is able to manufacture many crucial components, essential fatty acids are not on the list. Two important fatty acids are linoleic acid, an omega-6 fat, and alpha-linoleic acid, an omega-3 fat. From linoleic acid and alpha linoleic acid the body can produce nonessential fatty acids.

Omega-3 is one of the essential fatty acids produced by plants and may be present in animals who ingest a variety of foods like flaxseed, grass, hemp, leaves, nuts, seaweed, and walnuts. Omega-3 serves many important functions such as improving kidney functions, increasing metabolism, lowering triglycerides, and reducing the stickiness of blood platelets, thereby reducing the likelihood of blood clots. Docosahexaenoic acid (DHA) and eicosapentaenoic acid (EPA) are omega-3 fatty acids found in fish oil that have been shown to alleviate rheumatoid arthritis, enhance cognitive abilities, and reduce high levels of triglycerides. Researchers studied the diet of Eskimos who consumed high-fat diets, yet had remarkably low incidences of heart disease, which were attributed to diets high in omega-3 that reduced inflammation while promoting healthy heart functioning.

Good sources of omega-6 are present in unheated and unprocessed plant oils like corn, cottonseed, nuts, raw seeds, safflower, soybean, and sunflower. However, a little dab of oil will do ya because it can be pretty fattening and some oils may cause inflammatory reactions. Omega-6 provides some health benefits; however, studies show that an increase of omega-3 is needed to provide additional health benefits. To work optimally, omega-6 must be taken in proportion to omega-3 at a ratio of about 4:1. Many Americans consume omega-6 and omega-3 at a ratio of 20:1 respectively. When a considerable amount of omega-6 is consumed, more omega-3 is required in the diet or a significant reduction in omega-6 is required. The right amount of EFAs is important to the health of the body; however, eating too much or too little may cause health complications. Consuming insufficient omega-6 causes deficiencies while too much increases arachidonic acids (AA), which may cause inflammatory pain. In addition, consuming too much omega-3 may cause health complications like allergic reactions, low blood pressure, reduced clotting, and thin blood.

Cholesterol

Although cholesterol is necessary for good health, the body is able to make all that is needed. Blood cholesterol is sufficiently manufactured by the liver. Dietary cholesterol can be obtained from animal products like dairy, egg yolks, and meats. Plants do not produce cholesterol. Generally, foods that are high in cholesterol are also high in saturated fat. Some people try to take precautionary measures to reduce cholesterol by selecting moderately healthy foods like skinless white meat; however, this is not enough. The nutrients found in plant products have been found to reduce blood cholesterol while animal products have been found to increase blood cholesterol.

There are two different forms of cholesterol; the low-density lipoprotein (LDL) a.k.a. the bad cholesterol, and the high-density lipoprotein (HDL) a.k.a. the good cholesterol. LDL cholesterol coats and thereby narrows and hardens the arteries that nourish the heart and brain, increasing the likelihood that there may be trauma to the arteries and thereby may cause a life-threatening heart attack or stroke. On the other end of the spectrum, there is the more helpful HDL, good cholesterol. It is thought that HDL escorts cholesterol to the liver where it can be metabolized and excreted from the body, thereby alleviating some potential problems.

Triglycerides

Triglycerides are a form of fat that the body manufactures and also receives from food. Excess alcohol, limited physical activity, obesity, refined carbohydrates, saturated fat, smoking, and trans-fat cause the body to manufacture triglycerides. The body uses some triglycerides, but the rest are stored as fat. Excess triglycerides circulating in the blood plasma cause hyperglyceridemia, which is associated with cardiac disease, diabetes, high LDL cholesterol, and low HDL cholesterol.

Protein

One gigantic misconception about protein is that it has to come from meat. Protein is found in both plant and animal products. Proteins build enzymes, hormones, and tissues. Proteins also transport molecules and build, maintain, and synthesize new proteins.

Amino acids are the building blocks of proteins that build fluids, glands, hair, ligaments, muscles, nails, organs, and tendons. Amino acids are broken down into two groups: essential and nonessential. The body can manufacture nonessential amino acids from fats, carbohydrates, and other amino acids. However, the body cannot manufacture essential amino acids. Essential amino acids must be obtained from food. Protein production can be stopped or slowed without essential amino acids. In addition, there are three amino acids, glutamine, ornithine, and taurine that are nonessential until the body experiences disease or injury, at which point they become essential.

Essential amino acids may be categorized as complete and incomplete. Proteins that contain all amino acids are known as complete proteins while those low in one area are known as limiting proteins and others more deficient in amino acids are known as incomplete amino acids. Incomplete and limiting proteins may be coupled to create complete proteins, this is known as complementarity.

Those who prefer plant products can get all of their essential amino acids from plant products. There are many plant products that are quite rich in proteins; however, they have incomplete proteins and therefore don't have all nine essential amino acids in adequate quantities. Individually, plant products do not provide a complete source of protein like meat products, but they easily provide a complete source of protein when combined with other plant products.

Animal protein is considered high quality or complete protein because it contains all nine essential amino acids, which are similar to our body and easily absorbed. Essential complete proteins can be found in diary, eggs, meats, and seafood.

For many people, animal protein is a favorite part of the diet and for good reason, it is tasty and filling. Animal protein takes longer to digest than fats and carbohydrates; therefore, it may help you stay satisfied longer without the urge to eat, unlike refined carbohydrates. Animal protein is an important part of every meal, especially to diabetics because it helps metabolize sugars more slowly to keep blood sugar stabilized. Proteins eaten in combination with simple carbohydrates slow digestion, help regulate blood sugar, and help ward off hunger.

Animal protein is generally significantly fattier than plant protein. It is important to select lean meats. In addition, there are many lunch meats that are more than 90% fat free. To help reduce meat portions, try eating shredded, sliced, and diced meat.

While animal protein is an important part of your diet, over-consumption may promote the development of complications. The elimination of the nitrogenous waste created from eating animal proteins stresses the liver. Overindulging on animal protein can also cause insulin resistance. Insulin resistance impedes weight loss. Eating vast amounts of animal protein also increases the excretion of calcium. Experimental studies have found that consuming approximately 20% of one's diet from animal protein can promote the growth of cancer cells and cause liver complications. The good news is the negative effects of consuming too much animal protein are not produced from eating too much plant protein.

Protein is one of the most overindulged part of the American diet. Nutritional studies show that the body needs 2.5% of calories from protein daily. The World Health Organization (WHO) recommends that at least 5% of calories come from protein. The RDA recommends a diet of 9–10% protein to replenish one's daily supply. Many Americans routinely consume 11–21% of protein daily. Keep in mind that vegetables provide approximately 10% protein. Basically seven grams of protein is required for each 20 pounds. Therefore a 140 lb. person would require 49 grams of protein (one ounce = 28.35 grams) or about two ounces.

Hormones

Research has found evidence that hormones contribute to the body's ability to lose weight. Excess weight and body fat significantly disrupt not only hormones, but a series of functions, which further diminish the body's ability to effectively carry out processes and lose weight.

The good news is losing weight helps control hormones. Some of the important hormones related to weight loss include:

+ Leptin
+ Insulin
+ Gherlin
+ Serotonin

Leptin resistance is a hormone dysfunction that impairs the body's ability to effectively regulate appetite and metabolism. Under normal conditions, the body would be able to maintain its natural weight. If a few pounds were added, the body would suppress the urge to eat to return to its natural weight. When the body is adequately nourished it releases leptin to reduce hunger and increase the metabolism. However, this process is inhibited when the body does not receive adequate nourishment, like during dieting. Not only is the body not receiving adequate nourishment, but hunger often never subsides while the metabolism is reduced. Many diets are doomed before they start.

Cortisol is a hormone produced by the adrenal cortex of the adrenal gland. Cortisol plays a role in a variety of functions in the body such metabolism and the management of as fat, protein, and sugar. Without cortisol, the body would suffer a series of complications like serious fatigue, impaired immunity, and inability to cope with stress.

Insulin is the ringleader in the body's sugar circus. Insulin directs fat tissue, liver, and muscles to accept glucose or store it within the liver and muscles as glycogen. To lose weight, it is important to increase the cells' sensitivity to insulin.

Conclusion

As you can see, there is more to each food than meets the eye. When selecting foods to eat evaluation is paramount, not just the exterior, but the interior as well to ensure that it will nourish your body and promote your health.

Additives: What's the Deal? 8

INSTEAD OF ASKING what is added to refined and processed foods, it may be easier to ask what isn't added.
Foods are loaded down with the good, the bad, and the unimaginable
to create the prettiest, tastiest, longest lasting foods ever. Unfortunately,
many additives in foods can negatively impact your health. Drugs
are more thoroughly scrutinized than food additives, yet there is a
steady stream of dangerous drugs that enter the marketplace; what
else haven't we discovered about food additives?

Many foods are engineered to taste good—literally, the look, the
color, the smell, and the texture. In some dark laboratory filled with
bubbling test tubes and chemical formulas, there are scientists feverishly working to create the most delectable snacks with all kinds of
funky ingredients that will create the tastes we crave.

A smorgasbord of additives are routinely added to food and
drugs. Additives are used for a variety of reasons like to enhance
flavor, appearance, or shelf life. A few of the most common additives
include colors, emulsifiers, flavor additives, flavor enhancers like
MSG, preservatives, sweeteners, and synthetic vitamins. Although
most additives go undetected, some people are negatively affected
by additives in food. Additives have the ability to promote asthma
attacks, cancer, and neurological damage. Because of the synthetic

structure of food additives, it is difficult for the body to recognize and eliminate them.

Colors enhance the appearance of food. Color additives range from natural to highly unusual sources like FD&C No. 1, which is blue color, used in cosmetics, gelatins, hair dyes, and soft drinks. Emulsifiers like lecithin and polysorbate are regularly added to foods like pudding and salad dressing to keep the liquids from separating. Stabilizers such as alginates, derived from seaweed, creates creamy ice cream textures. Natural gums and starches thicken and increase the content of foods. Calcium carbonate is a texturizer that helps foods maintain firmness in cans. Sulfites are a preservative used to kill or impede the growth of bacteria. While preserving foods, sulfites cause the deterioration of some vitamins in food.

There are even chemicals present in the food packaging that the FDA does not require food companies to disclose. Do you really want to eat mysterious ingredients? Who knows what effect the multitude of chemicals will have on your body in the future? When possible, natural foods are a better choice.

Sugar

The world has an insatiable appetite for sugar, with more than 115 million tons produced each year. Sugar is a delightful addition to almost everything. Sugar tastes great and can put a smile on your face, but it also puts pounds on your body. The average American consumes approximately 158 pounds of sugar each year. Cake, cookies, and candy are not the only sugar packers. Even if you don't add sugar, it is hidden in many foods like alcohol, beverages, canned and frozen foods, cereals, dressings, energy bars, flavorings, meats, medications, peanut butter, sauces, and soups.

The scientific term for sugar is saccharide; however, it is known by many names and comes in many forms. Table sugar, a.k.a. sucrose, is a highly refined and chemically processed substance that involves physically compressing cane stalks or sugar beets, filtering and treating the remnants with acids to remove impurities, removing the molasses through centrifugation, then boiling, bleaching, and drying the product until the familiar white crystals known as sugar are created. Sucrose contains four grams of carbs and 16 calories per teaspoon.

Before the refining process, sugar does have some nutritional value, but it is stripped away until you get nothing but a sweet taste able to rot a good tooth with time. Sugar is a great additive because it increases bulk, while enhancing flavor.

Sugar contains no nutritional value, providing only empty calories. Empty calories without nutrients can results in malnutrition and obesity. Therefore, it is important to carefully review the label to determine the sugar content. When sugar is listed as one of the first five ingredients, it is a fair assessment to say that it is a major ingredient.

Like everything else in excess, sugar can cause health complications like the depletion of minerals, development of dental cavities, development of inflammation, and hormone imbalances. Reducing all forms of natural and artificial sugar is important to good health. Eating too much sugar impedes the absorption of vitamins and minerals and impairs the ability of white blood cells to rid the body of foreign pathogens, which depresses and weakens the immune system and may lead to a series of health complications. Inflamed, depleted, and weakened, the body is not able to carry out all metabolic functions, which promotes sickness and obesity, and increases the likelihood of contracting the cold, flu, and other ailments.

The body, being the ingenious creation that it is, prepares for the overconsumption of sugar with a steady stream of insulin to combat high sugar levels, which creates a hypoglycemic condition. Hypoglycemia is a serious condition because the brain requires a steady source of energy supplied by glucose, yet high insulin levels reduce the available glucose in the body, creating a strong urge to eat, often sweets, to increase the level of glucose, but a little is almost never enough and the vicious cycle continues.

Excess sugar increases the body's exposure to glucose and insulin, which causes internal bodily damage. Research studies report that sugar increases triglyceride levels and damages the heart. In order to reduce inflammation and triglyceride levels, limit the amount of sugar consumed.

Sugar addictions can be very strong because sweets produce a pleasurable sensation. Animals fed sugary drinks continued to sip copious amounts throughout the day. The incessant drinking did not curtail their eating, but rather increased it by 33%. Try the experiment with yourself. See how much sugary sweetness you chug versus plain ole H_2O.

Sugar withdrawals can cause very strong symptoms such as headaches, nausea, and mood swings. The only thing that may satisfy the intense urge is more sugar, but this triggers the cycle to continue over and over again. To end the cycle, transition to healthier foods and purge the sugary concoctions from your daily regimen.

The yeast, candida, loves sugar and uses it as a source of fuel inside the body. Candida causes bloating and water retention while straining the liver with its waste product acetaldehyde, which damages the body's tissues and organs, but candida is not the only sugar lover. Cancer cells love sugar too. Cancer cells utilize sugar as fuel to promote tumor growth. To reduce the likelihood of promoting the growth of cancer cells, it is important to reduce sugar consumption.

Some of the sugars you may encounter individually and within foods include, but are not limited to:

+ Brown sugar—sucrose with molasses syrup
+ Cane juice—sweet juice extract from sugar cane
+ Confectioner's sugar—powdered sugar
+ Corn syrup—a.k.a. high-fructose corn syrup (HFCS)
+ Crystalline fructose—processed fructose from corn

+ Dextrose—glucose or corn sugar
+ Fructose—fruit sugar
+ Fruit juice concentrate—generally flavored sugar water
+ Galactose—part of milk sugar
+ Glucose—a.k.a. dextrose
+ Honey—combination of fructose and glucose produced by bees and insects
+ Invert sugar—glucose and fructose: used in baked goods
+ Lactose—galactose and glucose
+ Maltose—malt sugar
+ Molasses—separated from raw sugar during processing
+ Darker and blackstrap molasses—provides small amounts of vitamins and minerals
+ Raw sugar—contains many impurities
+ Syrups—high-maltose corn, barley, malt, maple
+ Sucrose—table sugar refined from sugar cane or sugar beet
+ Sugar alcohols— mannitol, sorbitol, and xylitol
+ Turbinado—partially refined sugar: a.k.a. "raw sugar"

Fructose is found naturally in fruit and sometimes it is a good alternative to sucrose; however, it is just as calorie-intense as sucrose with four grams of carbs and 16 calories per teaspoon. Fructose does not have an intense impact on blood sugar, which is good news for diabetics. Fructose gives the allure of being healthier because it is from fruit; however, not all fructose is from fruit. Some fructose is chemically refined from modified corn and is packed with five grams of carbs and 20 calories per teaspoon, even more than table sugar.

High-fructose corn syrup (HFCS) has received a lot of flak, but many people believe that it is really not any more detrimental than cane or beet sugar; however, not everyone feels this way. HFCS was developed in 1968. Since the 1970s, HFCS has risen in popularity because it is cheaper and 40% sweeter than beet or cane sugar; it processes well, has a long shelf life, keeps food soft, produces a toasty coloring, and easily dissolves as a liquid. HFCS sweetens a gamut of foods like condiments, jams, juice, soft drinks, and wine.

Some people attribute the fattening of America to HFCS because its cheapness allowed for larger portions while not reducing profits. Too much of a tasty treat has not been good for everyone. Research shows that HCFS does not impact blood sugar levels in the same way as sucrose. HCFS is chemically refined from a starch and the body does not recognize the presence of HFCS, which may promote overconsumption and result in obesity.

Many people are interested in natural sugar sources like agave nectar. Although agave nectar provides more nutrients than sugar, it still contains five grams of carbs and 16 calories. There are reports of alternative sweeteners being passed off as true agave nectar; however, the alternatives are actually more similar to high-fructose corn syrup.

Although honey is a popular natural sweetener, it has stats similar to high-fructose corn syrup with six grams of carbs and 20 calories per teaspoon. Rice and barely syrups also have stats similar to corn syrup. There are many types of honey, which affect blood sugar differently. Most commercial honeys and syrups are highly refined and not so beneficial.

Stevia, a herb from South America, has been used for over 20 years in some Asian countries and for over a thousand years in South America safely and without any known negative side effects. The flavor of stevia is enhanced with fruit oligosaccharide, FOS. After a long wait, the FDA is not objecting to the public's use of stevia. Stevia is about 150 to 300 times sweeter than sugar with no calories and no effect on blood sugar. Not to mention stevia is inexpensive to grow and produce.

Yes, sugar causes a lot of complications, but that does not mean that you have to lead your life without sweetness. There are many foods found in nature that offer the sweet taste so many of us are fond of.

Natural sources of sweetness also supply nutrients like B vitamins, calcium, chromium, enzymes, fiber, folic acid, iron, magnesium, potassium, and protein. As an added bonus, researchers have found that reducing sugar and eating more fruits and vegetables improve the texture and the appearance of skin by reducing acne and wrinkles.

Sugar Alcohols

Sugar alcohols, a.k.a. polyols, are sweeteners, but aren't a sugar or artificial sweetener; they more closely resemble alcohols and are made from corn or wheat. Sugar alcohols do have a couple of advantages over sugar; they do not promote cavities and have fewer calories. There are a variety of polyols that are used in candies, chewing gum, and sugar-free foods. Some sugar alcohols you may see in the ingredients label include mannitol, sorbitol, and xylitol. In addition, sugar alcohols are not fully absorbed into the blood, so they do not cause significant spikes in blood sugar. But careful, too much of this quasi-good thing can cause bloating, cramps, diarrhea, gas, and a leaky bowel.

Artificial Sweeteners

Sugar sweetens and delights, but it has negative effects on the body, like blood sugar complications, fueling cancer, obesity, and tooth decay. The world's obsession with sweetness has left many searching for new sweeteners. After years of exploring and concocting, (mad?) scientists have developed different substances that emulate the sweet taste of sugar, without the same negative side effects. Artificial sweeteners seem like the perfect alternative to sugar. Sweet aficionados are willing to pay over 20 times more than the price of sugar for synthetic sweeteners to get the sensationally sweet taste without calories and guilt.

Artificial sweeteners are everywhere. Each year 7.5 metric tons of artificial sweeteners are produced and added to more than 6,000 foods and drugs. Artificial sweeteners are popular among dieters and diabetics. Table sugar causes a spike in blood sugar requiring insulin to help reduce the spike, but artificial sweeteners do not produce the same effects. Artificial sweeteners claim to significantly reduce calories, making them more desirable to those who want to lose weight.

Artificial sweeteners offer the same great taste as natural sugar with a sliver of the calories; however, there is a price to be paid for the highly sought after sweetness, but the price just isn't monetary. Artificial sweeteners are highly complex chemical concoctions, most of which were discovered by scientists experimenting with toxic chemicals. There are mounds of damning information about artificial sweeteners; however, they still continue to be in demand.

Artificial sweeteners promote acidic conditions within the body, which can promote illness. When the body becomes too acidic it withdraws minerals such as calcium from the body, which promotes osteoporosis.

Although many people turn to artificial sweeteners to save calories and lose weight, many researchers believe that consuming artificial sweeteners promotes sugar cravings. Not to mention, many artificial sweeteners actually contain bulking agents similar to sugar. Dextrose, a combination of glucose and maltodextrin, is a common bulking agent. Why not just eat table sugar? In addition, many people who consistently consume artificial sweeteners often eat more than they would if they had not consumed them.

Research data from animal studies shows that high consumption of artificial sweeteners is correlated to an increase in cancer. Experimental studies also have shown that animals given artificial sweeteners develop brain tumors and seizures. However, to assuage fears, researchers attribute the increased development of cancer in animals to physiological differences that exist between the animals and humans. Physiological differences aside, there has been an increase in incidences of cancer among diabetic artificial sweetener users; however, the risk is not considered significant. In addition, shortly after the introduction of artificial sweeteners there was a marked increase in the development of brain tumors in the US.

In search for the perfect sweetener, many natural and artificial sweeteners have been identified. There are several artificial sweeteners currently used across the world; however, due to their negative side effects, not all are approved for use in the US. Worldwide, some of the most used artificial sweeteners have been saccharin, cyclamate, aspartame, sucralose, acesulfame-K, and neotame. Each one is a chemical concoction that has the potential to cause physiological complications and each one has its own tale of troubles.

In a research lab in 1879, a researcher working with dangerous chemicals accidentally discovered saccharin, the first artificial sweetener. One hundred years after saccharin was made publicly available, studies revealed that it promoted bladder disease in rats. This prompted the FDA to issue a warning label on saccharin, but after additional studies the warning label was removed; not because it was safe, but the risk was not highly significant.

Dulcin was the next artificial sweetener made available to the public, but a long-term study during the 1950s found it to be toxic, even at small doses. The next accidental lab creation was cyclamate. Cyclamate had less of an aftertaste than saccharin, was water soluble, cheaply produced, and had no calories. Cyclamate was used for almost two decades in combination with saccharin in Sweet 'N Low until evidence surfaced that it caused cancer in mice if consumed in vast amounts. Cyclamate was banned by the FDA in 1969; however, it is still available in other countries.

Aspartame, alitame, sucralose, acesulfame-K, and neotame were the next major artificial sweeteners to be introduced to the public. Acesulfame-K, a.k.a. Sunette, was accidentally discovered in 1967. Acesulfame-K was approved for limited use in 1988 and additional uses in 1998. Acesulfame-K contains methylene chloride. In addition to cancer, acesulfame-K may cause headaches, organ damage, and visual complications.

The artificial sweetener aspartame, which is commercially known as Equal is an FDA approved sugar substitute. Aspartame is present in numerous foods, especially foods promoting low and no sugar. Nonetheless, Equal is an equally bad option. Equal contains the amino acid phenylalanine, and at high doses it can increase the possibility of depression, seizures, and schizophrenia. The methyl alcohol within aspartame can form formaldehyde within the body. And when combined with carbohydrates, aspartame can have negative effects on the brain by reducing the production of serotonin, which is necessary to good mental health.

Studies on aspartame reveal the development of a series of complications including, but not limited to: arthritis, autoimmune diseases, atypical facial pain, birth defects, brain tumors, confusion, diabetes, dizziness, epileptic attacks, headache, memory loss, tremors, and damage to the organs, genetic material, nerves, and the immune system.

In 1997 neotame was approved as a tabletop sweetener, and five years later it was approved as a general sweetener. A little dab will do yah, considering neotame is seven to thirteen thousand times sweeter than sugar. Unlike aspartame, neotame does not break down into phenylalanine, which is toxic to people with PKU. Neotame contains small amounts of aspartic acid and methanol, and collectively these two can be hazardous to your health.

Sucralose, also known as Splenda, is the number one selling artificial sweetener with over $187 million in sales in 2005. Although Splenda is often promoted as a close cousin of sucrose, table sugar, it is actually a chemically chlorinated compound full of poisons like arsenics, heavy metals, and methanols. Sucralose is 600 times sweeter than sugar with a hefty price tag of $450 per kilo. Is it artificial sugar or what? Sucralose doesn't have a bitter metallic aftertaste like other artificial sweeteners. Sucralose was inadvertently discovered in the quest for a new insecticide, so how safe could it be? Like everything else, if the poisons are in a small amount the product is approved by the FDA, but is it really safe?

There have been incalculable complaints made regarding artificial sweeteners to the FDA, more than any other food additives, yet little has been done. The most alarming part of the history of artificial sweeteners was the doubts of their safeness—suspicions were swiftly cast aside. Some artificial sweeteners were removed from the market, but a considerable length of time passed while the dangerous concoctions were available for everyone's everyday consumption.

The irrevocable data needed to clearly define artificial sweeteners as safe is non-existent. Much of the data about artificial sweeteners was collected from small scale human studies, studies on animals with physiological differences, or random studies pertaining to the properties of artificial sweeteners. Moreover, the studies are generally completed by the artificial sweetener manufacturer, which is clearly a conflict of interest. Nonetheless, the initial discovery of most artificial sweeteners was from a scientific experiment in search of poisons, which inadvertently happened to be sweet. Needless to say, this doesn't seem like the ingredient that should be added to morning coffee, even if it does have fewer calories and a flat line effect on blood sugar.

There is no solid evidence that demonstrates artificial sweeteners will improve weight loss; in fact there is evidence that artificial sweeteners stimulate hunger. Studies have shown people who regularly consume artificial sweeteners have hunger pangs soon after consuming artificial sweeteners, which can have a negative effect on weight gain. Artificial sweeteners are a bad idea. Skip the artificial sweeteners and limit your sugar or sweeten with fruit.

Caffeine

Many people enjoy the stimulating effect provided by caffeine. Sometimes we crave it and sometimes it's just something extra that is not given a second thought, but it deserves a second thought. Caffeine comes in a variety of forms like chocolate, coffee, energy drinks, over-the-counter pain medication, soda, and tea. Caffeine affects everyone differently, but as a mild stimulant it has the ability to increase blood pressure, heart rate, metabolism, and urination. In addition, caffeine affects cortisol levels, promotes dehydration, impacts digestion, and reduces the body's ability to release toxins. Caffeine may also cause constipation and ulcers.

Caffeine has a diuretic effect on the body, causing the body to expel liquid and promote dehydration. A dehydrated body is not a peak performing body. As a stimulant, caffeine inhibits the production of melatonin in the brain for up to nine hours and thereby inhibits sleep. Sleep deprivation leads to increased cortisol production, which interferes with glucose metabolism and creates insulin resistance, all of which aggravates heart disease and may impede weight loss. Caffeine also taxes the liver, which may impede the liver's ability to break down fats and may slow weight loss.

Caffeine contains approximately 30 different acids that creates acidic conditions within the body. The body's attempt to neutralize the acids promotes osteoporosis. Studies show that caffeine causes genetic abnormalities within plants and animals. Pregnant women who ingest caffeine may cause their fetus a series of problems including, but not limited to: low birth weight, spontaneous abortion, or other damage. Caffeine has negative effects on the brain including disturbing the enzymes utilized in memory making.

Everyday consumption of caffeine can lead to the body's dependence on it. Eliminating caffeine from your diet can be difficult. Caffeine is sometimes hidden in different items like chocolate, over-the-counter medications, and supplements. While the body has a continual supply of caffeine, it is fine; however, when the caffeine disappears, the body begins to go through the withdrawal process and may initiate excruciating migraine headaches.

Kicking the caffeine curse can be challenging, but you can start off by reducing the amount of caffeine you drink daily with each drink, for instance most tea contains less caffeine than most sodas and coffee. Once you have gradually reduced your intake of caffeine you are more prepared to quit; this will help reduce the withdrawal effects that you may experience. Caffeine essentially has no taste, so you won't be missing the flavor. Some may miss the jolt provided by caffeine; however, a good diet will quickly replace any jolt.

There are many good alternatives to caffeinated beverages such as decaffeinated green tea and water. Decaffeinated green tea has stellar qualities including the ability to protect against allergies and cancer while also decreasing blood pressure. However, be careful, some decaffeinated drinks are highly acidic, which is not good for the body.

Condiments

Condiments add pizazz and make foods tastier, but too many additives can make good foods bad and impede weight loss. Some condiments can add hundreds of calories to your meals, so whenever possible leave your food in its birthday suit.

Ketchup is a good place to cut the calories. Although made with tomatoes, ketchup is heated, processed, doused with sugar, and sprinkled with chemicals. Mayonnaise is another calorie-packed condiment. Luckily, you do not have to cut the mustard. Although most condiments are generally full of fat and calories, mustard is not.

Butters, oils, and sauces make foods taste great, but they are generally fattening. There are ways to enhance flavors without adding tons of calories. Herbs and spices are a great way to add flavor while keeping the calories low. Different combinations of herbs can transform meats and vegetables into brand new foods that may become your favorites. Not to mention, the beneficial effects of eating naturally grown herbs and spices. Check out all the herbs and spices to see what flavors you may fancy.

Instead of soaking your food in sauces, put them on the side. Sauces and gravies are brimming with sugar and calories. You can savor the flavor while saving some calories. Instead of smearing and lathering bread in butter; use healthy oils like olive or canola sparingly. While both oil and butter are heavy on the calories, butter has seven grams of saturated fat while olive oil has less than two grams per tablespoon.

Salt and Spices

Sodium, more commonly known as salt, is a notorious little mineral. It has built up quite the reputation; however, it is an important part of the diet. Only 1500–2300 mg, a teaspoon or less, of sodium is needed by the body per day. Less sodium is needed for individuals that have high blood pressure or have reached middle age. Overindulging in sodium can lead to high blood pressure.

There is a fine balance of vitamins and minerals that must be present within the body to keep it working optimally. It is important to monitor your salt consumption to avoid any adverse health effects. Sodium helps regulate the fluids in the body. When there is increased salt intake, the body takes in more water. When salt is reduced, additional water weight may be lost, thereby promoting weight loss.

In addition to sodium, calcium, magnesium, potassium, and zinc help to regulate the fluid within cells. These elements help promote good osmotic balance and blood pressure. Potassium works in tandem with sodium within the body, so it is important to consume sufficient amounts of both minerals. These minerals are found in a well-balanced diet; however, if your diet is inadequate, vitamin and mineral supplements can provide the nutrients needed. In addition, large amounts of salt have the ability promote calcium excretion.

Salt is everywhere like canned foods, preservatives, and refined foods. Some inconspicuous foods may contain large amounts of sodium without the strong salty taste, so beware. Condiments like ketchup, mustard, pickles, olives, and soy are high in sodium. In addition, certain styles of food also contain high amounts of sodium such as au jus, broth, Chinese, pickled, and smoked.

Some people sprinkle salt on their food out of habit; however, moderation is key; taste your food to ensure that the extra salt is necessary. Salt is not the only addition that can add flavor to food. Instead of sprinkling salt, try adding flavor to your food with herbs, natural fruit juices, and spices. Cutting back on salt may seem like a chore; however, by gradually reducing the amount of salt used, reductions can be accomplished in no time.

Although sea salt is frequently promoted as the healthy salt alternative, sea salt and table salt have virtually the same properties. The only differences that exist between sea salt and table salt are taste, texture, and processing. Sea salt is developed by evaporating seawater. The source of the seawater contributes to the presence of minerals, taste, and texture. Table salt is from highly refined underground salt deposits. The refining process extracts all trace minerals. However, unlike sea salt, table salt contains iodine, which is essential to the thyroid.

Spices like cinnamon, cloves, and nutmeg improve the body's ability to metabolize sugar while enhancing the flavor of food. Other spices like bay leaves, cayenne, coriander, dry mustard, and ginger may help manage blood sugar levels, reduce inflammation, and increase the body's temperature and metabolism.

Conclusion

While there are many additions that can enhance the flavor of food, the refined and processed additions come with negative effects to the body. If possible, try to enjoy food with as little refined additions as possible to do the least amount of damage and reap the most rewards.

Thirsty? 9

DRINKS HAVE COOL COLORS, sugary sweetness, fizzy carbonation, and enticing flavors, but you pay a price for the delight. Drinks can be a bad investment of calories. You may not even realize you are drinking away your daily calories. Have you ever noticed how many times you'll reach for a tasty flavored drink versus how much you grab water? Sweet drinks and sodas increase the likelihood of overeating and devouring excess calories.

Most sweet drinks contain a mountain of calories and a molehill of nutrients; even juice is only marginally better than soda with its loads of calories and sugar. Some fruit drinks sprinkle in a couple of vitamins and nutrients to promote a healthy façade, but a dash of vitamins does not supersede the presence of artificial flavoring, preservatives, and sugar. Even sports drinks are not much better than the average fruit drinks.

When indulging in your favorite beverage, check out the calories per serving size and the number of servings presence. Today's beverage sizes usually supply two or more servings. If you take sugar in your coffee or tea, consider that one teaspoon of sugar adds 16 calories. Every calorie counts. While you're on your journey to a leaner, healthier you, remember that calorie-charged drinks can grossly affect your waistline. Don't waste your calories; eliminate or reduce the calories imbibed from drinks to enjoy your food. Water is the best selection to rehydrate.

Alcohol

"Your body is a temple, but keep the spirits on the outside."
— UNKNOWN

There are mixed messages floating everywhere about alcohol. Drink alcohol; it's good for you. Don't drink alcohol; it's bad for you. Well, there is truth in both of the statements depending on a number of factors like your gender, type of alcohol, quantity of alcohol, and frequency of alcohol consumption.

Alcohol is a sedative that provides some temporary benefits like expanding blood vessels and reducing the risk for blood clots. Although relaxing and sometimes tasty, alcoholic beverages are chocked full of carbs and calories. Alcohol promotes the release of endorphins, which may cause addiction and dependency.

Many alcohols contain additives called sulfites, which inhibit bacterial growth while extending the expiration date. However, for approximately one in every 100 people, sulfites may cause a range of negative sides effects like breathing difficulties, hives, migraines, sneezing, swelling of the throat, and in the rare and extreme case, death. Alcohol without sulfites will have a label that states "No Sulfites Added" or "NSA." In addition to sulfites, cancer-causing agents such as urethane are present in some alcohols, even the organic versions.

Alcohol is notorious for its empty calories; it has tons of calories and zero nutrients. Depending on how much you drink, cutting back on alcohol may reduce mega-calories. Moreover, consumption of alcohol may stimulate cortisol production, which may lead to increased weight gain and promote fat storage. Not to mention, alcohol may increase hunger for up to a week.

Serving Size	Calories
12 ounce bottle of beer	150
8 ounce mixed drink	150
5 ounce glass of wine	100
100 ounces of water	0

Alcohol is absorbed through the lining of the mouth, throat, stomach, and small intestine. While in the stomach, alcohol is metabolized by an enzyme known as gastric alcohol dehydrogenase (ADH). Men produce more ADH than women; it helps to quickly break down alcohol and reduce the inebriating effect. Because women produce less ADH, alcohol remains in the female system longer and has a more inebriating effect. The liver can detoxify about one drink (6–12 ounces of beer, five ounces of wine, or one ounce of liquor) per hour, but this can vary from person to person.

Moderate amounts of alcohol can increase levels of HDL (good cholesterol), improve digestion, and improve blood circulation. Research studies report that individuals who drink two to four alcoholic beverages per week are less likely to experience coronary or circulatory complications. Researchers also found that men with this pattern of alcohol consumption developed fewer cases of cancer over 10 years. The positive results diminished for men who drank more than two alcoholic beverages per day. On the other hand, the results are somewhat different for women. Although alcoholic beverages may improve circulatory and coronary conditions, there is an increased risk for breast cancer among women who drink three to nine alcoholic beverages per week.

Wine boasts some significant benefits including the ability to diminish the risk of cancer and cardiovascular disease. The skin of grapes contains resveratrol, which studies show to have anti-inflammatory properties, as well the ability to reduce cholesterol. Drinking wine three to four times per week may reduce a man's risk for heart disease; however, the same amount may increase a woman's risk of developing breast cancer by over 40%.

While a small amount of alcohol may be beneficial, too much alcohol can have negative effects such as cardiovascular disease, depression, high blood pressure, immune system suppression, impotence, increased production of free radicals, increased risk of cancer, infertility, liver and brain damage, strokes, and reduced absorption of vitamins, minerals, and other nutrients.

Alcohol may also alter the effectiveness of prescription and non-prescription drugs, dehydrate the body, suppress the immune system, and thereby increase the likelihood for infections and illness.

Numerous studies have shown that alcohol provides health benefits with an unhealthy diet; however, consuming alcohol is not without risks. To reap the most benefits, it is best to eat a healthy diet while avoiding alcohol. If alcohol is part of your diet, carefully consider the negative outcomes that may ensue. A drink a couple of times during the week may provide some benefits to your health; however, the benefits of drinking alcohol are not profound enough for a nondrinker to start drinking

Dairy a.k.a. Liquid Meat

Dairy is big business in the US. To entice consumers to drink milk, the dairy industry creates pretty packages, assorted flavors, and optimal temperature storage. To promote its products and increase sales, the dairy industry spends hundreds of millions of dollars. Milk does a body good; or at least that is what one of the milk industry's multimillion dollar campaigns reports. We've also learned milk helps you grow and build strong bones, but there are some negative factors that aren't as well known. All that glitters is not gold, and all the hype about milk is just not true. Although milk is considered a beverage, its contents beg to differ; it is more like a liquid version of meat. Milk and meat have different physical properties, yet they have many similar effects on the body, which is perfectly logical considering milk and meat are from the same source. Milk also contains the same contaminants as meat like growth hormones, pesticides, and steroids. Therefore, all of the undesirable effects from eating meat can occur from just drinking milk.

Dairy advertisers would have you believe that milk is the best thing under the sun, but in reality milk contributes to more problems that it alleviates. An eight ounce glass of milk is packed with about five grams of saturated fat, lactose, 150 calories, pesticides, and hormones. Milk is extremely fattening, and should be consumed moderately. Forty-nine percent of the calories in whole milk are from fat. Even 2% milk contains 35% of its calories from fat. Why call it 2%? Because its 98% fat free by the water weight—slick trick. It is important to remember that the purpose of milk is to nourish a newborn calf to a 2,000 pound cow, so it's reasonable to believe that it is fattening. Milk-based products are fattening too. Cheese is a wonderful topping to almost everything. It tastes so yummy because 70 to 80% of its calories are derived from saturated fat; even the low-fat options still contain 50% fat. In addition, almost all cheeses contain pesticide residue.

Drinking a glass of milk requires the enzyme lactase to dissolve the sugar, lactose, which is found in milk. As we age, the production of lactase is significantly reduced, inhibiting the body's ability to digest milk, which does not create favorable conditions in the intestines. Some people are sensitive to milk and may feel bloated or gassy after drinking it. Over 50 million Americans have a lactase deficiency, which impedes their ability to break down lactose and causes a series of symptoms including abdominal pain, diarrhea, gas, and nausea.

Milk consumption also increases the likelihood of the following complications: autoimmune diseases, multiple sclerosis, osteoporosis, prostate cancers, and type I diabetes. The consumption of milk has been correlated to a series of additional health complications such as allergies, anemia, arthritis, attention deficit disorder, autism, cancer,

Crohn's disease, colic, depressed immune response, diabetes, ear infections, fibromyalgia, headaches, heartburn, heart disease, indigestion, irritable bowel syndrome, joint pain, and obesity.

And forget about the gentle milk maiden milking the cow. The 10 pounds of milk a cow would normally produce in one day is just not good enough, so cows are given growth hormone to crank it up to about one hundred gallons per day. Metal contraptions yank milk out as fast as it can flow, causing infections, sores, and pus to flow right in the milk, which necessitates pasteurization to lower, but not eliminate the amount of bacteria in milk while also increasing shelf life. Pasteurization also destroys nutrients. In the US, vitamin D is routinely added to milk.

Estrogen, progestins, androgens, and insulin-like growth factors are some of the hormones that you'll be downing in a glass of milk. Elevated levels of hormones have been linked to the increased risk of cancer. Numerous research studies report that men who consume high amounts of dairy significantly increase their risk of developing prostate cancer.

Osteoporosis is a disease that affects more than 28 million Americans. Osteoporosis is the gradual loss of bone density that increases the likelihood of bone fractures. In the US, there are over 1.5 million fractures per year, of which 300,000 are broken hips. Statistics report that one-quarter of broken hip sufferers die within one year due to complications.

The best solution to eliminate or alleviate osteoporosis is a well-balanced diet that includes a variety of vegetables rich in calcium, as well as strengthening exercises to enhance muscles and improve stability to prevent falls. The truth is that multiple research studies have not found milk to prevent osteoporosis; however, studies have found that milk actually promotes osteoporosis by creating acidic conditions within the body. The body strives to neutralize acidic conditions by leeching minerals from the bones, thereby resulting in osteoporosis. In addition, it has been found that countries like the US, Finland, and Sweden that consume the most animal products, have the highest rates of osteoporosis.

With about 300 milligrams per glass, milk is a good source of calcium. The dairy industry would have everyone believe that it has a monopoly on calcium; luckily, milk is not the only source of calcium. In fact, there are several vegetables that contain even more calcium than a serving of milk. Vegetables that contain a good source of calcium include: beans, broccoli, cabbage, calcium-fortified orange juices, certain cereals, grains, greens, low-fat yogurt, kale, okra, seaweed, soybean products, and watercress. If you're looking for nutrients, milk is not the answer.

If you fancy milk, remember it is important to limit your consumption. Also be mindful of all of the products that you eat that may be milk-based. Ingesting copious amounts of dairy products also hinders the absorption of iron, which may result in anemia.

On the flipside, there are some studies that show dairy can promote weight loss and reduce body fat. However, with all of the concerns regarding fats, hormones, intolerance, sugar, and toxins surrounding cow's milk, it might be time to investigate some of the alternatives. Milk and milk-based products are not your only option. There are a plethora of new, healthier products that have a texture and taste that resembles milk without all of the side effects.

Alternative Milks

Nut, rice, and soy milks represent alternatives to drinking milk; they do not contain animal products and are suitable for vegans. Alternative milks do not contain lactose, so they are good for anyone who is lactose-intolerant. Some alternative milks may be thickened with carrageenan and tapioca. If you don't like one, try another. The tastes vary by brands, flavors, and types. Most alternative milks have very little natural fat and are often fortified with vitamins and minerals. Alternative milks are available in grocery and health food stores and can be a substitute for everything with milk like: cereal, creamers, frozen dairy treats, ice creams, pudding, smoothies, and other recipes.

Rice Milk

Rice milk has little protein and carbohydrates and may be fortified with essential vitamins. Rice milk is packaged in paper containers and may be found in the refrigeration aisle to prevent spoilage; however, it may also be in aseptic containers, which do not require refrigeration before opening. Generally, rice milk has a shelf life of one to two weeks once opened. Shipping costs, low demand, and subsidies paid to American rice growers increase the cost of rice milk.

Rice milk can easily be made at home. To make rice milk, boil a cup of rice of your choice with four cups of water, blend the rice until it is finely shredded, and strain the mixture with a strainer, nut bag, or cheesecloth to remove rice. Flavor and sweeten to taste with vanilla, chocolate, cinnamon, spice, or rice sugar. The rice may be cooked an additional time with tree nuts or spices to make the flavor of your dreams.

Nut Milks

A variety of nut milks can be used to create a high protein milk alternative for anyone who is allergic to cow's milk, a vegan, lactose intolerant, or trying to reduce calories. Many types of nut milks are available in stores. Some commercial nut milks may contain milk products like casein, which is not tolerated well by everyone. However, nut milks, like almond milk, are easily made at home with a blender.

To make nut milk, mix approximately one part nuts to four parts water, one part nuts to three parts water, or one part nuts to two parts water, reducing the ratio of water makes creamier milk.

A variety of additions like honey, dates, or spices can enhance the flavor. Raw recipes avoid cooking while utilizing soaking. Nuts can be soaked for a day prior to blending. Boiling facilitates the milking process. Boil the liquid and nuts for a few minutes, blend, and strain the mixture. The nut pulp can be refrigerated, sprinkled on cereal, added to cookies, eaten with raisins, or baked in goods. Nut cheese can also be made from the nut pulp as a substitute for dairy cheese.

The nutritional value of homemade nut milks is difficult to determine. Nuts vary in fat content; however, they are generally much lower or similar to dairy milk. In general, nut milks are usually fairly high in protein, but they are not generally an adequate source of calcium, unless they are fortified.

Soy Milk

First developed in Asia, soy milk is a beverage made from soybeans. Soybeans have high concentrations of isoflavones, which are believed to be healthy. Many vegans and vegetarians prefer soy milk to cow's milk, as do people with lactose intolerance. It may take some time to acclimate to soy milk; it has a slightly beany flavor. Flavors like chocolate, strawberry, vanilla, and other substances can enhance flavor to ease the transition from cow's milk. Review soy milk's label carefully to determine if artificial substances and sweeteners have been added, which may diminish the quality with excess calories. Some commercial soy milks have stabilizers to increase their shelf life.

Soy milk is available in many grocery stores and restaurants; however, it can be made at home by hand or with a soy milk machine. A soy milk machine can also be used with nuts and other beans. To make soy milk, soak dried soybeans in water for at least three hours or more, blend mixture to a slurry, and boil to enhance flavor. Cool, strain, and enjoy.

Juices

If you're thinking about drinking tons of the wonderfully flavored commercial juices off the shelf of your local grocer to reap the benefits of juicing—forget about it. Although many fruit juices claim they are made with natural fruit juice, most do not contain much nutritional value. Fruit juice is not the nutritional equivalent to fruits and vegetables, despite all the claims from advertisers. Most juices are a combination of flavoring, sugar, and water. Fruit juices contain a significant amount of sugar, which the liver will most likely convert to fat. Commercial juices are generally devoid of any nutritional value because of pasteurization. While extending the shelf life and guarding against bacteria, pasteurization destroys the enzymes and nutrients found naturally in juice. After pasteurization, all that is left is a sweetly flavored juice. Consuming copious amounts of juice may increase dental cavities while adding unwanted pounds.

On occasion, some juices are unpasteurized in an effort to keep the nutrients and enzymes; however, this can be dangerous if there is a serious overgrowth of bacteria in the juice, which can cause severe sickness. Juicing and eating fresh fruit right after peeling or juicing provides the most nutrients.

Juicing

With thousands of different combinations of fruits and vegetables, you're sure to find some favorites. Unlike the sweet flavored water at the grocery store, juicing provides nutrient-rich, vitamin-packed juice that can provide you with many benefits. The high water content of juice makes it a great hydrator. Citrus fruits like grapefruits, lemons, limes, and pineapples are good solvents that help purge the liver and the gallbladder. Wheatgrass provides sweet juice that is packed with nutrients including chlorophyll, which is a chemical found in the chloroplast of plants known for its healing effects on infections, sores, and wounds. Wheatgrass is pretty sweet, but it can be combined with other vegetables to enhance the flavor.

Keep in mind that as soon as fruit is picked, it begins to lose its nutrients and the countdown is still going after you juice your fruit, so drink it or refrigerate it soon after juicing. Juice can remain in the refrigerator for a few days, but refrigeration only slows, not stops deterioration. Time and exposure to air degrades the nutritional content found within juice. Freezing juices will extend the life of the juice; however, freezing will also destroy some of the nutrients.

Although juicing is a good way to get nutrients, additional nutrients and fiber can be obtained from eating whole unprocessed fruits and vegetables. Juicing condenses fruits and vegetables by removing the beneficial fiber, creating a big glass of nutritious, yet calorie-intense liquid. The pulp extracted from juicing fruits and vegetables does not have to be discarded; it can be used in breads, fertilizer, muffins, and soups.

The juicing-challenged fruits include:

Avocado	Banana	Coconut	Peach	Papaya
Apricot	Cantaloupe	Honeydew	Plum	Strawberry

Some fruits, like berries, are not recommended for juicing because they do not produce a significant amount of juice. Some fruits have too much pulp that cannot be separated from the juice like bananas and melons. Although fruits like papaya are not recommended for juicing, they can still be enjoyed by blending the pulp with water or another juice. In addition, you can drill through the shell for coconut milk.

Smoothies

A smoothie is a fresh, quick, delicious, and nutritious drink ready in just minutes. Smoothies can be a great way to have a drink, snack, or a meal. Depending on your personal preferences and dietary requirements you can sweeten your smoothie naturally with fruit or unsweeten it with vegetables. Blend different combinations of fruits, ice, ice cream, juice, milk, sherbet, vegetables, water, and yogurt. Be careful, some additions may add significant calories to a potentially low-calorie treat.

Soda

Over the last 50 years, soda has increased immensely in popularity. Soda garners 25% of the US beverage market. Over 600 cans of soda are produced per person each year. Soda contains exorbitant amounts of sugar and calories while being devoid of nutritional value. Extra pounds can be shed easily by replacing soda with water.

The fizzy carbonation that tickles our taste buds also taints the insides of the body. Carbonated drinks contain phosphoric acids, which weakens bone mass, depletes the calcium stores within the body, promotes the development of osteoporosis, and may cause gas.

Diet soda is not any better. Unlike non-diet sodas sweetened with high-fructose syrup, diet sodas rely on artificial sweeteners to give them the same sweetness of non-diet soda that people love, which may result in health complications.

Coffee

Many people enjoy the caffeine jolt, the flavor, and the aroma of coffee; however, theses perks come with a toll. The caffeine in coffee is mildly addictive and can keep you coming back for more. Too much coffee on a daily basis may produce heartburn, insomnia, irritability, shakes, ulcers, withdrawal symptoms in the absence of coffee, and bone loss, which also increases the risk of broken bones.

But the news about coffee is not all bad. The research concerning coffee consumption shows some positive effects, but like everything else, coffee is good in moderation. Some of coffee's redeeming qualities include:

+ Reduces suicide—coffee may serve as a mild antidepressant. Studies have shown a 50% reduced suicide rate among coffee drinkers.
+ Reduces the risk of developing kidney stones—may be attributed to the diuretic effect of coffee that may inhibit the growth of kidney stones.
+ Reduces the risk of developing gallstones—caffeine impedes cholesterol crystallization and stimulates the gallbladder, which may hinder gallstone development.
+ Reduces risk for type II diabetes—results from the Nurses' Health Study and Health Professionals' Follow-up Study show that those who drank five or more cups of coffee per day had less incidence of diabetes.

Tea

Tea, the world's second most popular beverage, next to water has been enjoyed for thousands of years. Tea offers a wide variety of health benefits including reducing the risk for cancer, gallstones, kidney complications, and obesity.

Most teas contain approximately half the caffeine content of coffee. While most coffee contains 85 milligrams of caffeine, tea contains about 40 milligrams. Numerous studies have validated the benefits of tea. Black, green, oolong, and white tea leaves from the *camellia sinesnis* tree contain antioxidant polyphenols. Consuming four to six cups of black, green, oolong, and white tea daily reduces the risk of a developing a variety of cancers such as gastric, esophageal, ovarian and skin.

Tea is loaded with flavonoids, which reduce cancer, cavity causing bacteria, and cholesterol. Green tea has catechins. Catechins are antioxidant flavonoids. Studies have found that drinking three glasses of tea per day can increase metabolism and reduce body weight and waist circumference.

Polyphenols are not the only valuable ingredients lurking in the tea. Tea contains a variety of vitamins and minerals, all of which have beneficial health effects like:

+ Delay aging
+ Prevent blood clots
+ Lower cholesterol levels
+ Reduce the risk of cancer
+ Impede the growth of tumors
+ Stimulate the immune system
+ Protect against mutagenic agents
+ Protect against high blood pressure
+ Protect against viral and bacterial infection
+ Protect cells from the normal, but harmful, oxidative stress
+ Improve the functions of the digestive and excretory systems

Herbal teas are a bouquet of flowers, herbs, roots, spices, and other plant parts, but unfortunately they do not have the same healing effects as the *camellia sinensis* leaves; however, herbal teas are known for their ability to relax and calm.

Water

Although any drink can satisfy thirst, there is no substitute for water. Popular beverages like alcohol, coffee, energy drinks, sports drinks, and tea may have additives, caffeine, and sugar, which may dehydrate and stress the body. Water is the most essential nutrient required by the body. You can live without food for weeks, but go a couple days without water and you'll wake up on the wrong side of the dirt. Water constitutes a large portion of the body, about 50 to 70% and more than 80% of the brain. Water does incalculable good for the body. Water cushions, bathes, and lubricates internal structures, hydrates cells and organs, flushes away toxins, facilitates digestion and metabolism, sends electrical messages, regulates body functions and temperature, reduces the risk of cancer, and sustains blood volume.

While resting, thankfully, the body is still at work. Therefore, it is important to hydrate the body well before you go to sleep and when you wake up. Many factors affect the body's requirement for water including activity level, disease, food, weather, and weight. Throughout the day the body loses water through breathing, defecating, excretion, evaporation, and perspiration; it is important to continually replenish the water that is lost. Everybody is different and has different water requirements, but a good rule of thumb is one-half of your weight in ounces of water for replenishment. Consuming sufficient amounts of water is even more important in certain situations like eating high protein meals, exercising, experiencing high blood pressure, hot environments, and taking medication.

Your daily diet will affect the amount of water that is required. All sources of water count toward your daily requirement. A diet of meat and bread will require more water than a diet of fruits and vegetables. Fruits and vegetables contain a substantial amount of water, which helps fulfill the daily water requirement.

Thirst is not a very good gauge of how much water is needed by the body. By the time thirst is triggered, water levels within the body may be very low. Water is especially important as we age. Studies have shown that as we grow older, our sense of thirst is reduced. Rehydration does not occur immediately. It takes cells a period of days to become replenished. Although many people rely on the pale color of urine to validate a sufficient consumption of water, this is not always an accurate indicator.

When rehydrating, it is important to replenish electrolytes. Electrolytes include chloride, potassium, and sodium, which can easily be found in sports drinks or a well-balanced diet. Electrolytes help the body transmit electrical impulses, facilitate digestion, and regulate cellular activity.

The sensation of thirst and hunger are often confused. Before eating anything, drink a glass of water to determine if you are thirsty or hungry. Without adequate hydration, one may be compelled to eat more to fill the void generated by dehydration. In addition, water is a calorie cheap alternative to gobbling up goodies.

It is important to select good hydrators like water. Inappropriate hydrators will exacerbate dehydration and may cause additional complications. Vasopressin is a hormone that helps the body conserve water in a shortage. However, alcohol inhibits vasopressin, thus intensifying dehydration.

Good hydration helps prevent physiological damage. Researchers report that drinking sufficient amounts of water may reduce the risk of cancer by 50%. Moreover, water has the ability to reduce the excess cholesterol deposits within the arteries. Water is especially important to asthmatics. When the body is consistently hydrated, it reduces the production of histamines, which are part of the brigade that helps defend the body against foreign invaders or pathogens that triggers allergic reactions like a runny nose and watery eyes.

Dehydration is highly stressful to the body and may cause a series of problems like dizziness, fatigue, fever, headache, increased pulse, nausea, organ failure, shortness of breath, and ultimately death. Without adequate hydration, your circulation will slow. Droughts in the body's water supply also impede the body's ability to remove toxins, which may contribute to the accumulation of body fat, cellulite, and toxins. Water helps remove the waste from metabolic processes. Insufficient water inhibits healing and toxin removal and slows digestion. Water facilitates the excretion of metabolic waste and toxins and helps return the body's natural balance. Over time, if water is consistently short and the toxins aren't reduced, the body can turn against itself and develop autoimmune diseases, which may be deadly.

Dehydration may elevate blood pressure. When the body is dehydrated it takes more pressure to hydrate cells and circulate blood throughout the body to provide oxygen and nutrients to cells for metabolic activity. Without adequate hydration, the cells within the body will constrict to conserve water loss, which will cause swelling and increase in blood pressure. Blood cells are composed of 94% water; being dehydrated decreases the water content of blood and thereby impedes metabolism. If dehydration is the reason behind high blood pressure, you would most likely be given a diuretic, which will increase urination and thereby exacerbate dehydration.

The body is quite flexible and at times initiates unimaginable actions to take care of itself, which ultimately may lead to greater problems. Moreover, some researchers believe chronic dehydration may be the culprit behind many illnesses and diseases. The body strives to be slightly alkaline at an optimal pH around 7.35. When the body is more acidic from ingesting foods like soda and meat, the body attempts to leech out elements to reduce acidity and return the body to a more alkaline state. Water washes away acidity, returning the body to its optimal pH.

The body has the ability to accumulate a wide variety of toxins and remnants of substances such as uric acid, which may cause joint pain. It may sound too simple to be true; however, water has the ability to alleviate some pains and illnesses. Cells continually work and over time accumulate acidic waste. Without adequate water to remove toxins and waste, acidic conditions may cause pain. Painkillers alleviate pain, but do not fix the real problem. Water has the ability to neutralize the acidic conditions and eliminate the pain, without any of the harmful side effects caused by drugs.

Acidic conditions in the brain may have a negative effect over time and lead to disease. Adequate water supply to the brain is vital because its cells cannot regenerate, unlike other parts of the body like the liver. Dehydration may compromise the integrity of the blood-brain barrier. When this happens, any residual solid material may result in the formation of plaque, which has been notoriously linked to ferocious neurological disorders such as Alzheimer's, multiple sclerosis, and Parkinson's.

Water is also an important part of digestion and elimination. When water is scarce, the body attempts to reabsorb every droplet of water before defecation. Insufficient hydration may result in little brown pellets instead of a brown banana in the porcelain pool, which is a sign that you need more water. If you can't go, then you may be constipated. Constipation can lead to some serious conditions such as diverticulitis, hemorrhoids, and polyp formations that may lead to cancer.

Water may not excite your taste buds like many of the other drinks available; however, all of the good that it can do for your body should increase its appeal. If you ever grow tired of water's taste, enhance the flavor without mega-sizing the calories by adding fruit or natural fruit juice.

Apple Cider Vinegar

Commercial apple cider vinegar is aesthetically pleasing, pasteurized, filtered, and refined; unfortunately, these processes have destroyed the healthy, endogenous nutrients. Unrefined raw apple cider vinegar is cloudy, with a brown tinge, and packed full of vitamins and minerals like beta-carotene, calcium, chlorine, fluorine, iron, magnesium, pectin, phosphorous, potassium, sodium, and sulphur. Unrefined apple cider vinegar provides benefits that:

+ Reduce bad cholesterol
+ Help regulate blood pressure
+ Reduce free radicals damage
+ Eliminate toxic waste from the body

+ Reduce fungal and bacterial infections
+ Strengthen hair, weak fingernails, and brittle teeth
+ Break down fat to promote weight loss
+ Help extract calcium from fruits, vegetables, and meat
+ Dissolve uric acid deposits around joints to relieve pains

Apple cider vinegar can be used in a variety of ways to enhance the healthiness of foods and drinks. Try the following:

+ Marinating meat
+ Sprinkling on salad
+ Using as a dipping sauce
+ Adding two tablespoons of vinegar to a glass of water

Conclusion

There are many sensational selections that can tickle our taste buds and satisfy thirst, but they also have the ability to add excess calories and impede weight loss. To maximize your weight loss efforts, select drinks that will hydrate the body and build on the momentum of a good diet.

PART III

How to Lose Weight in the Real World

How Do I Succeed on a Diet? 10

Eating Habits and Hunger

> *"One should eat to live, not live to eat."*
> — Cicero, Rhetoricorum LV

Food is at the center of so many events it is no wonder why food is sometimes overused and abused. In many cultures, celebrations center around tasty and often fattening foods. Although food is festive, it may be necessary to use alternative ways to heighten festivities that will not minimize your weight loss effort and undo your progress.

Making good decisions about what to eat is one of the most important parts of your diet. You can restrict enough calories to lose weight, but if the body does not receive adequate nourishment the desire to eat may be overwhelming.

Eating right is a culmination of many factors like what you eat, how much you eat, when you eat, and how you eat. Generally, one food is not responsible for the overall quality of a diet. The overall diet has to do with all of the foods eaten on a regular basis that holistically impacts your health and weight.

Dietary studies show that many people tend to overeat when they have skipped meals or are angry, depressed, emotionally distraught, lonely, or tired. When food is used as a mood enhancer, it is only a temporary solution that requires constant replenishment, to the detriment of your health. It is important to deal with hunger and feelings as they emerge so that you will be able to control situations. Dealing with the source of issues may be more productive in the long run, rather than superficially improving any situation in the short-term. If you are upset, clean, cry, dance, exercise, read, scream, shop, talk, walk, yell, or get a punching bag. Experiment with different activities to find the solution that works best for you.

There are many people that experience different ailments like depression, fatigue, and headache, who try to self-medicate with food. If there is a problem, figure out the cause; don't just treat symptoms with food. Individuals with hypoglycemia may continually eat to ward off headaches and feeling ill; however, medicating on food is not the answer. For many hypoglycemics, low blood sugar causes the body to want, even crave junky carbs. Refined carbs satisfy many cravings, but they are not always the most nutritious. Unlike complex carbohydrates and proteins, which take longer to digest and break down, refined carbohydrates are easily digested and satisfy hunger quickly, but hunger returns sooner rather than later. This ravenous cycle of cheap carbs is quickly crushed with a more satisfying and nutritious diet.

Many people ward off the uncomfortable feeling associated with hunger by eating before hunger sets in. Eating before true hunger sets in can be problematic because the body may store the extra calories as fat.

Carefully consider the size of your meals. It is easy to consume a day's worth of calories at one sitting: a tasty fried appetizer, an entrée, an appetizing beverage, and a dessert, can easily add up to more than a day's calories. Despite how much is eaten at the previous meal, most people want to eat again in three to four hours. So don't use all of your calories at one meal. Carefully consider all of your meals throughout the day to be sure that you do not ingest excess calories.

It is easy to overeat, especially when the food is good. Decide beforehand how much you are going to eat. You control your diet; your diet does not control you. Always pay close attention to how much you are eating when focusing on other tasks like playing games, socializing, watching TV, or working. It is easy to turn on the automatic pilot and mindlessly munch away. Eating from a bag can also be deceiving. Bags can camouflage supersized snacks. Separate your food to a small plate to see exactly how much you are eating and try to refrain from seconds. Foods like chips, cookies, and peanuts may trigger more eating. Your tummy may plead for another after another, even after you promised yourself you had your last one 10 bites ago.

To curtail excessive eating, grant yourself more, but later. It is better for your body to eat small meals; therefore, space your meals and snacks out over time. Sometimes as little as 20 minutes will help you recognize fullness and give you the power to say, "I'm full." You can also drink water, eat fruits and vegetables, and exercise. Taking additional measures will help ensure that you don't overeat.

Water should be taken at the first sign of thirst, but it should also be the first thing you reach for at the first sign of hunger. Many people confuse the first signs of thirst as hunger. Water is an essential part of the diet and should be consumed throughout the day to promote a well-functioning body. Water can help fill the stomach and facilitate digestion while decreasing the volume of the food consumed. You may just find out that you are not hungry at all and saved yourself some calories. It might be the solution that you have been looking for.

Daily Meals

"We never repent of having eaten too little."
— THOMAS JEFFERSON

Although this may seem like a given, it is important to eat adequate amounts, even when dieting. Some people try to maximize their diet by severely reducing their calorie consumption to accelerate weight loss; however, this may cause malnutrition and a slow metabolism, both of which may impede weight loss efforts. When the body doesn't receive nourishment it doesn't just use up the extra stored fat; it might eventually get around to doing that, but the first thing that it does is conserve energy by slowing down the body's metabolic processes. The last thing you want to do while dieting is slow down your metabolism, so keep the food rolling. If you really want to try a radical diet to lose weight, eat tons of fruits and vegetables every day. Throw in a couple of ounces of meat to cover all of your bases.

Daily eating can turn into a smorgasbord; there are so many wonderful foods to eat, but variety can be the downfall to a diet. Studies show that individuals who consistently eat the same type of food for at least one meal per day lose more weight. Now this doesn't mean that you have to eat the same food all day long, but the same meal for breakfast, lunch, or dinner throughout the week.

Enjoying one consistent meal each day can eliminate the randomness of meals that may contribute to overeating. Consistency also eliminates the guesswork; that means no quick stops or unhealthy alternatives to your planned healthy meal. A consistent meal can be fruit or oatmeal for breakfast or a salad, sandwich, or soup for lunch. Planned meals provide some wiggle room for you to enjoy a variety of foods within the same category to make your diet enjoyable.

The culturally established three meals a day just doesn't work for everybody. Hunger often strikes before meals arrive. In lieu of the three meals, four or five small meals may be a better solution; however, a series of little meals may pack more calories than intended, so be careful when eating many small meals throughout the day; the calories will add up and may add to the problem instead of the solution. Eating large meals may cause the body to consume more calories than it can use at one time, thereby forcing it to store the excess calories as fat. The body can more easily digest small meals versus large meals.

Breakfast

Some people aren't especially hungry in the morning and prefer to skip breakfast. Others look at skipping breakfast as an opportunity to save on calories. These are not good ideas; it's not called the most important meal of the day for nothing. Studies show that people who eat breakfast are more successful at losing weight and keeping it off. Skipping meals puts the body into starvation mode, telling the body to ration energy in times of famine. Breakfast ends your nightly fast, while kick-starting your metabolism. You could skip breakfast altogether, but you'd prolong your fast and keep your metabolism in low gear. No one said that you have to have bacon, eggs, grits, pancakes, toast, and a cup of orange juice; any little thing will do like a piece of fruit, a serving of fiber-packed cereal, or an egg.

A good way to ensure that you consume your daily allotment of fruit is to have it for breakfast. Fruit supplies energy in the morning to start a day off right. Studies reveal that people who eat breakfast perform better than those who don't. The best way to beat powerful cravings is to begin the day with a healthy breakfast. Eating in the morning may help reduce binging and excess hunger throughout the day. Eating fruit for breakfast may also satisfy cravings for sweetness while improving your health. Unlike processed food that may have you feeling heavy and sluggish, fruits can provide you with a jolt unlike anything else. In addition, most fruits need little or no preparation—just cut, peel, or bite and voila! Breakfast is served.

Yogurt can be a great breakfast and a good snack. Some yogurts have good bacteria and promote improved gastrointestinal health by reducing or eliminating constipation, diarrhea, H. pylori infections, inflammatory bowel disease, and lactose intolerance. Yogurt provides a variety of benefits such as protein, about nine grams in a six ounce serving, along with calcium, B_2, B_{12}, potassium, and magnesium.

Plain yogurt is the best way to go. Although tasty, flavored yogurts are more than likely loaded with sugar and offer less benefits to your health. Buy the plain yogurt, but it doesn't have to stay plain for long. There are many additions that you can mix in with yogurt to enhance the flavor and make it a tasty treat. Berries, flaxseed, and nuts are a couple of the additions that can make yogurt a delightful snack.

Fiber and protein are important parts of breakfast. For breakfast, eat whole grain cereal or oatmeal with at least five dietary grams of fiber per serving; some cereals contain significantly more with over 20 grams of fiber per serving. Whole grains can be paired with fruit to increase the nutritional value while satisfying hunger longer than just fruit alone.

Lunch

After you eat your fruits at breakfast, lunch is another opportunity to improve your health with vegetables. Dark greens are packed with nutrients that can give you the energy to endure the rest of the day. Salads and veggies for lunch help get your required servings of vegetables out of the way for the day, so you know that you have taken care of your body. For those of you that have to have a little meat to make a meal A MEAL, you can easily add a variety of meats to salad to give it what you crave while getting the nutrients your body needs. Beef, ham, salami, seafood, turkey, and tuna all can enhance a salad to make it a wonderful lunchtime meal.

There are so many wonderful reasons to pack a lunch from home. Depending on your schedule, you might not get enough time to really enjoy lunch. You can save time and avoid feverishly searching, deciding, going, getting, and eating your lunch. Phew! You can take the time that you have saved to relax and enjoy your lunch. Bringing your lunch from home can also save you money. Hey, who knows what you like better than you? Pack, eat, and enjoy.

If you have been eating well all day you can guiltlessly enjoy your dinner. What a great feeling!

Dinner

"Eat breakfast like a king, lunch like a prince, and dinner like a pauper."
— ADELLE DAVIS

So what may a pauper's dinner consist of? Something that is light, not going to weigh you down, make your stomach turn, and your esophagus burn. Many people believe that they have rightly earned and deserve a good dinner after the daily toils and troubles, but it often leaves millions searching for relief provided by over-the-counter pills that mask the indigestion brought on by dinner. Food should never leave you with feelings of discomfort and despair.

A light dinner can be just as satisfying or even more so than a hearty dinner, without the guilt, heartburn, indigestion, and pain. Some choices for light meals include, but not limited to:

+ Fruit
+ Soup
+ Salad
+ Cereal
+ Beans
+ Vegetables
+ Sandwiches
+ Whole grains
+ Three to four ounces of lean meat

To eat or not to eat late at night? That is the question. While sleeping, the body needs to rejuvenate and rest, not work on digesting your last meal. Therefore, to facilitate digestion it is important to eat at least two to three hours before you go to sleep. The extra movement during waking hours aids digestion and prevents indigestion. Shortly after falling to sleep, growth hormone is released. Growth hormone is needed for the body to perform optimally. Eating close to bedtime may impede the release of growth hormone.

Dinner is an opportunity to share a meal with your family and expose them to healthier choices. This is especially important to children. Eating habits can last a lifetime. Be sure that the foods you expose your children to are the foods that will promote their health.

Snacks and Cravings

"Opportunity may knock only once, but temptation leans on the doorbell."
— Unknown

You may still hear your mother's voice ringing in your ears not to spoil your dinner, but do it! The lapse time between meals can be considerable—making you quite hungry—maybe even famished. It is easy to overeat when you are extremely hungry. You can avoid overeating by having a planned light snack in between meals. It is important for you to eat when you are hungry; losing weight is not about starving, but making good decisions that will promote your health and weight loss.

A familiar scenario for many people—you have just ate and you're satisfied, but snacks are calling your name. Yoo-hoo! How about a little snack-e-poo? Hunger is a powerful force, it can bring all activities to a halt to be satisfied, which makes perfect sense; hunger is the force that supplies the body with the energy, so it may override everything to get what it needs. But sometimes, cravings are disguised as hunger. It is imperative to control cravings. If you know that you've had enough, but hunger just won't leave you alone, try drinking a glass of water or eating fruits and vegetables. Refocus on something else—get up and get busy.

Most of us could generally go for something tasty, even right after we've eaten and we know that we shouldn't. You have to learn to recognize true hunger. Not the feeling of, "I could go for that." Just let that feeling pass right by. That feeling gets no snacks. True hunger resembles a deep grumbling that comes three to five hours after eating—that is the feeling that we feed. It is vital to stop eating once your hunger has been satisfied. If you listen to the directions of your taste buds, you may continue eating long after your hunger has been satisfied because food often tastes so good we just take bite after bite. Satisfying taste buds can add pound after pound.

Our favorite foods are usually high in sugar, fat, or something else not so nutritious. Can you have your cake and eat it too? Test your will power—will a little dab of chocolate satisfy you? A small portion assures you that you aren't missing out on anything while satisfying your craving. Instead of trying to eliminate your favorite foods, which may intensify your cravings into a gargantuan monster, have a little piece. A little piece may satisfy your craving and help you move on. But this is only if you can; you know your strengths and weaknesses.

If you know that one bite will transform you into a sugar-craving banshee, just resist the urge. Don't wallow in the deep dark pit of temptation. Those pesky cravings will hang on you like a monkey on a banana, but you have to resist. Stay strong. Get away from the food or start an activity that will help you focus on something other than the food that will thwart your progress.

Although packaged snacks are convenient and tasty, try to keep them off your snack list. Refined carbohydrates have too many negative ingredients and may easily contain hundreds of calories in a bite sized snack. Good snack selections include fruits, vegetables, and nuts. Review the label to find extra ingredients lurking in the package that may thwart your weight loss efforts. Avoid all products that contain high-fructose corn syrup, partially hydrogenated oils, refined flour, natural and artificial sugar, and saturated and trans-fats. Also, be careful of the quasi-healthy treats like protein bars. Protein bars seem like a good, healthy idea, but a closer look at the ingredients may reveal chemicals, preservatives, and sugar.

Dried fruit is a good snack, but the drying process destroys some of the nutrients, removes water, and packs more calories per ounce than fresh fruit. Nuts are a great, tasty snack and they're a good source of protein. Nuts are little and may seem like a light, treat, but six to ten is quite enough because they can pack a lot of calories. Cracking nuts immediately before eating them will slow you down and ensure they are fresh, not rancid. Fruit is an excellent snack; granted, fruit is not as filling as a T-bone, but there are ways to combat this dilemma like eating more fruit, whole grains, or a slice or two of lean lunch meat.

Desserts

"Forget love, I'd rather fall in chocolate."
— UNKNOWN

Mirrors, mirror on the wall, what makes m f el best of all?

Desserts can be a considerable source ries. A slice of cheesecake can have c 1,000 calories. It is a good idea to reduce the size of desserts by sharing or saving part of it, or better yet, have a piece of fruit. Fresh fruit is a good alternative to high-calorie, nutrient-deficient desserts. Fruit provides delightf sweetness, reduced calories, and nutrients as an added bonus.

Digestion

Don't dig your grave with your own knife and fork.
— ENGLISH PROVERB

There are multiple factors that contribute to good digestion, which include, but are not limited to: adequate hydration, exercise, good nutrition, and limited portion size. Excess food taxes the entire body by stealing energy and promoting fatigue.

Crazy diets cause poor digestion, but what else could be expected with limited food? Whether it is the special liquid concoction of the week or anything under the stars except carbs. One of two things is going to happen, you're either going to be as backed up as rush hour traffic or as loose as a jezebel in a brothel. Crazy diets don't make for a happy pooper.

Food takes approximately 39 hours in women and 31 hours in men to digest and pass out of the body. Digestion times vary from person to person depending multiple factors. After ingestion, the boluses of chewed food make quite the journey through approximately seven meters of narrow canals. The type of foods and beverages ingested greatly affect the passage of poop. To ensure a smooth and easy passage, reduce refined carbohydrates, dairy, and meat, while increasing natural unrefined carbohydrates and water. A good diet and sufficient hydration will help alleviate most elimination issues.

Fibers like barley, brown rice, corn, fruits, oats, rye, vegetables, and whole grains are important players in digestion. Increasing dietary fiber may alleviate constipation within hours or days. As an added bonus, when stools pass easily, less straining is necessary, which may help relieve hemorrhoids. Being continually constipated can lead to another pot of problems, including, but not limited to: bad breath (something's brewing down below), hair loss, headaches, and heavy menstrual bleeding.

Digestion is facilitated even more by thoroughly chewing each bite of food. Chewing breaks down food and extracts the nutrients, especially roughage. Larger pieces of food are more difficult for the body to break down and extract nutrients.

Slowly eat your food; if you eat fast you may overeat. In addition, if you eat too fast you may cause a series of discomforts to yourself like farting, hiccups, or gas from swallowing too much air while eating, so take it easy. The slower that you eat, the less you may eat. It takes time for the body and brain to recognize fullness, so give your body the time that it needs. Eating slowly helps digestion and promotes the absorption of nutrients.

We often consume more calories than our bodies need. You're not a teddy bear; don't stuff yourself. If you eat until you feel stuffed, you've really eaten too much. Consuming too much food causes the stomach to distend, compress, and suffocate other internal parts like the aorta, arteries, and the diaphragm. Many people associate being full as the point to stop eating; however, it's best for your body and your health if you stop eating when you're about 70% full. Research studies conclude that people who refrain from overeating live longer and healthier lives. Your body can only process so much food at one time. When excess food is consumed, the body decides to store the rest as fat. It may feel unnatural to stop eating before you are full, but you'll get used to it and your body will thank you for it. Eating less may alleviate indigestion, promote digestion, and help you lose weight. Enjoy the feeling of not being stuffed. Eat till the rumbling below subsides. The hunger pangs will be gone, and of course you could eat a little more, but you're satisfied. Eating till you are full may cause indigestion, stretch your stomach, make you feel guilty, and reduce the progress that you have achieved.

Eat well during the day and save the lighter meals for dinner. Eating the heaviest meals early during the day may facilitate food digestion, keep you fuller longer, and reduce snacking. Many people move less at night, which may impair digestion, contribute to indigestion, and disrupt sleep and rejuvenation.

Notice the difference in how you feel with every bite you eat, the good and the bad. Eating should never make you feel sick or uncomfortable; if it does, it is time to change your diet. There are millions of Americans who consume foods that make them sick daily; they seek relief in the form of heartburn and indigestion medication. This is great for the drug companies, but not great for your body. Medications, alcohol, allergens, and non-steroidal anti-inflammatories (NSAIDs) irritate and inflame the stomach's lining and reduce the production of gastric acids that break down food and facilitate digestion. If the food that you are eating is giving you indigestion, then you need to eat different food. There are tons of great foods available that will not make you sick or uncomfortable.

Plan

> *"Obstacles are those frightening things that become*
> *visible when we take our eyes off our goals."*
> — HENRY FORD

In the US, temptation is lurking around every corner, literally. The 99¢ specials at every fast food restaurant, the birthday cake at parties, the candies at the checkout counter, the sugary breakfast treats in the employee lounge, the free samples at the grocery store, and the home cooked food from friends and family. Not to mention, there are over 170,000 fast food restaurants and over three million vending machines stocked with goodies ready to squash your resolve in no time flat. It is no wonder why it is so difficult for many people to actually have the restraint against the barrage of food, but it can be done.

Hunger is going to strike, so prepare for it. When you are unprepared for hunger, you are more likely to select quick and easy remedies like fast food, vending machines, and convenience stores packed with chips, cookies, and candy, but you already know this will magnify the issue. Driving to and from work and around town can present a challenge if you are tempted by restaurants and fast food joints, but there is an easy solution. Always keep a snack prepared. Having a nutritional snack readily available will remove the need to fall prey to unhealthy choices.

There are many perils on the road to good health. Planning your meals will help you stay strong against food landmines ready to jackhammer your resolve. Many factors control what we eat like convenience, cravings, mood, and time, but we often do not give enough consideration to which foods will be in the best interest of our bodies. All meals need careful consideration; your health is worth the extra effort. Busy lives and schedules encourage many people to make nutrient-deficient food selections. A solid plan identifying when and what to eat can help you stay strong and reduce temptations. Giving into temptations can quickly undo any progress achieved.

Starting new activities can be fun and exciting, especially preparing for them. Preparing puts you on the road to success. Depending on what you want to exclude from your diet, you may need to give away, donate, or throw away food from your kitchen. If you leave dastardly remnants around, it may be easy to fall off track. Get off to a great start by cleaning out your pantry.

Nothing is more frustrating than to be on a diet for a significant period of time without success. Without a plan to guide you to success, slipups can easily occur. In order to have a well-balanced diet it is important to plan meals. The body has many requirements that aren't always satisfied with one type of food. Having a plan removes the stress from eating. Plan nutritious meals, and your diet will take care of itself and decrease the likelihood of grabbing a quick fix from fast food dives and vending machines.

There may be times in social settings when the food arrangements may be unknown or you do not have 100% control; however, you can still stay in charge by eating beforehand. If your hunger has already been satisfied—make a deal with yourself that you are not going to eat or sample anything, which can work out great if the food really isn't that good and you don't want to hurt the host's feelings. You can graciously say, "I've already eaten and I'm not hungry, but it looks and smells great!" If you can't or don't want to eat beforehand, use your knowledge of food; evaluate the food options that are available and make the best choice, this can be very empowering. You can also bring an item. The host may appreciate the offer and you will have a good option in lieu of unsavory foods.

When transitioning to a healthier style of eating you may not be familiar with the healthy foods you like to eat, and that is OK. Sample different foods until you find what you like. You may not have even discovered your favorite foods until you give yourself the opportunity to explore new foods. Keep an open mind when trying and implementing healthier foods into your diet. Given a reasonable chance, you may develop a passion for healthier foods.

Grocery Shopping

Some people avoid the grocery store like the plague because of the lines, extra time, and inconvenience. Eating out is just so much easier, but when you're eating healthy, the grocery store may be a necessary evil to get fresh fruits and vegetables to nourish your body.

Going to the grocery store hungry is just like taking a sugar fiend to a candy store; it's dangerous, don't do it. When you're hungry, cravings may control you and hurt your efforts. In the event that you are hungry in the grocery store, snack on fruit to stay in control of the cart.

It is hard enough to survive temptations with the lure of food on every street corner; your home should be a safe haven that promotes your health. The great thing about your home is—if you don't fill it with tempting foods, you'll be less likely to eat them. Only buy foods that will promote your health. When in doubt, leave it out. If you don't buy it, you won't eat it.

Do your grocery shopping with a list. A list will help you focus on the foods that you need and may help you think less about the foods that you may be trying to avoid. Select foods that are going to keep you nourished for breakfast, lunch, dinner, and a snack or two in between; don't leave any of your meals to chance. Preparing for meals will armor you against cravings, temptations, and unhealthy options.

Try to avoid buying separate foods for family and friends; it may ruin your diet. It will not hurt your family and friends to improve their eating, at least while they are in your presence, but if they truly fancy unhealthy items that are not on your menu, keep their goodies in a separate location—out of sight, out of mind.

When you are shopping, compare foods to ensure that you are getting the best product. Depending on the manufacturer, one product may have more of an unhealthy ingredient than another. This is good information to know when you are making decisions about what to eat, but if you don't look, you won't know.

Labels

The 1990 Nutrition Labeling and Education Act was created to provide consumers with information to help them make informed dietary decisions. A lot of information can be learned from the Nutrition Facts chart like:

+ Total calories
+ Sugar (in grams)
+ Calories from fat
+ Proteins (in grams)
+ Nutritional content
+ Total fat (in grams)
+ Trans-fat (in grams)
+ Dietary fiber (in grams)
+ Saturated fat (in grams)
+ Cholesterol (in milligrams)
+ Total carbohydrates (in grams)
+ Major ingredients listed in order from most to least

Only a few refined foods escape the labeling process like:

+ Coffee and tea
+ Deli and bakery items
+ Spices and flavorings
+ Restaurant-prepared items

Carefully reviewing food labels can help you make better dietary decisions. Even if you don't eliminate anything from your diet, it is important to know what is in everything you eat and how much you consume per day. Just the mere knowledge of the ingredients may influence what you decide to eat. Some ingredients to watch for include: chemical additives, HFCS, partially hydrogenated oil, natural and artificial sugar, refined flour, and saturated and trans-fats. Based on your knowledge, determine if the ingredients are right for you.

Labels are a good tool to help you cautiously review food contents; however, blind faith in labels is not prudent. Don't be comforted by the promise of labels; remain vigilant about the perils of foods. Many labels have double entendres, seeming to say one thing, but really meaning another. Review nutrition labels for the breakdown of the contents and calories. Some labels promise you a delight without the fright, but there is generally a catch. Who knew you would have to be a sleuth to determine the truth when reading labels, as if eating right isn't hard enough.

Good carbs, bad carbs, and net carbs; what's the difference? The carbs used by the body are known as net carbs or impact carbs. Net carbs may or may not be listed on the Nutrition Fact label; however, when they aren't, you can calculate them.

Total carbs – (total grams of fiber + glycerin + sugar alcohol) = net carbs

It is not enough to read the serving size on the side of food containers; you have to go further. For instance the label may state 100 calories per serving. That is not the end of the story. Next, look at the number of servings. This is especially tricky when the portion is so small it may appear to be only one serving, like a bag of five cookies. That definitely seems like one serving, but look further and the label reveals two cookies per serving at 100 calories per serving. After reviewing the label, you realize that those five cookies will add 250 calories, not the initial 100 calories you saw at first glance.

Although serving sizes may vary, they are generally the same for products in the same category. This allows for easy comparison of different items. Nonetheless, the amount of the serving size may not reflect a normal portion size. In fact, serving sizes are often minuscule, but this allows for the calories per serving size to be small and often misleading.

The percent daily values found on the nutrition label has the potential to provide important information concerning carbohydrates, fats, minerals, proteins, and vitamins to help you make good dietary decisions; however, the percent of daily values on packages may be inaccurate for you. Recommendations are based on a 2,000 calorie diet. Unless you are burning a lot of calories every day, a 2,000 calorie per day diet is probably too many calories to consume to help you lose weight. Keeping that in mind, it may be necessary to do a couple of mathematical computations to make the percent daily values relevant to you.

The label law requires foods to meet certain requirements to contain specific terminology. For instance:

Term	Meaning
High	One serving has 20% or more of the daily value for a specific nutrient
Good	One serving has 10–19% or more of the daily value for a specific nutrient
Light (lite)	Referring to calories, fat, or salt. One-third fewer calories, 50% less fat, or 50% less sodium than the regular product
Low-calorie	Forty calories or less per serving
Low-fat	Three grams or less per serving
Low saturated fat	Less than .5 gram of trans-fat or one gram of saturated fat
Low-cholesterol	Twenty milligrams or less
Reduced saturated fat	Twenty-five percent less trans-fat and saturated fat in comparison to the regular version
Calorie free	Less than five calories per serving

Term	Meaning
Fat free	Less than .5 grams per serving
Trans-fat-free	Less than .5 gram trans-fat and .5 saturated fat per serving
Cholesterol-free	Less than two milligrams of cholesterol or two grams or less saturated fat
Sodium free	Less than 5 milligrams of salt / sodium
Sugar free	Less than .5 grams of sugar
Reduced sugar	Still has sugar—generally 25% less than the regular version, still has about 75% of the regular sugar content
Low fat and no fat	May have more sugar
Made with whole grains	Only has to have a speck
100% whole wheat	Could mean it has a speck of 100% whole wheat
Multigrain	Could be refined grains
Whole grain	May be blended with refined, processed, or enriched products
Blends	Not 100% whole grains
Good source	Eight grams of whole grains per serving
Excellent source	Sixteen grams of whole grains per serving
Supports health	Any food can claim this; however, a stronger claim is "May reduce the risk."

Many products tout low and no fat, as if all fat is bad. Don't turn your worry meter off just because the label says "fat free." The fat-free label gives the illusion that food is healthy and you can eat all that you want, but that is not true. Just as much caution should be given to fat-free foods, perhaps even more because the label forgot to mention that more sugar and carbs are generally added to enhance the flavor of fat-free food, so that they remains somewhat tasty. Fat is also sometimes replaced with chemical compounds that resemble fat or protein compounds. The fat-free version generally has the same or slightly fewer calories. The food industry has a vested interest in keeping consumers coming back for more, and low and no calorie foods are appealing to most consumers. It is easy for consumers to eat more if they believe that food is healthy with limited calories. Low and no calorie foods lull the masses into a false sense of comfort when they believe foods do not pose any negative effects to their body while their health deteriorates right before their eyes.

There has been a large trend to reduce the fat in foods over the last couple of decades; yet the results of research studies show that Americans have been getting plumper and plumper, even though food has less fat, so the fat content of food is not the entire problem. There are no research studies that conclude that the fat content of foods is the primary reason for weight gain. What does make people gain weight is excessive calorie consumption. Once food is consumed, a portion is immediately used for energy, a portion is transformed to glycogen, and the rest is stored as fat. Fat contains nine calories per gram, which is more calories than both protein and carbohydrates; however, not all fat is bad. A little fat is needed to help with a variety of functions within the body. Remember—a little, too much fat can cause health complications.

Serving Size

> *"To lengthen thy life, lessen thy meals."*
> — BENJAMIN FRANKLIN (1706–1790)

Would you like to get something extra by paying nothing extra? Heck, yeah! Most Americans are always in the market for a good deal, and that is how many fast food offers appear—Get tasty treats like hamburger, fries, or fried chicken, for just a buck. Make it big for a few cents more! If it sounds good to you, you're not alone. Many Americans are enticed by the offer of mounds of food for a few dollars, in lieu of going home to cook after a long day at work. Although the idea of cooking after work does not seem attractive, you get what you pay for. Skip the values. It is very tempting to pay a couple of cents extra or twice as much food, but it just may be the downfall of your health and diet. Sometimes it's just better to get what you need or less. Fast food seems like a good deal at the time, but the price is a lot heftier than the 99¢ price tag that hangs from many specials. The price is generally your health.

Fast food portions are big, cheap, and tasty, which is turning out to be a dangerous combination for many Americans. Everyone wants more bang for the buck, but the bang has a bad effect on the body. Over the last couple of decades, serving sizes have significantly increased. During the 1950s a normal beverage serving size was eight ounces. Nowadays, a child's drink at McDonald's is 12 ounces and a large is 32 ounces, even 44 ounces at some fast food restaurants. The gargantuan sizes may be quite the deal, but the calories packed in the beverage can shoot your daily calorie count through the roof while providing limited nutrients and satisfaction. Although serving sizes may vary, on the average serving sizes have grown dramatically. For example, take a look at the tremendous average growth over the years:

+ Cookie sizes have tripled
+ Pasta portions have doubled
+ The original Hershey bar was .6 ounces, now its 1.6 to eight ounces
+ Cokes were 6.5 ounces, now they're 20 ounces with 250 calories
+ Bagels were three inches and 150 calories, now they're six inches and 350 calories

With portion size out of control, it is hard to know exactly how much to eat, especially when you hear your mother's voice in your ear saying "you're not leaving the table until your plate is clean." Remember, you're not getting an award if you clean your plate.

Amazingly, the new massive sizes are now standard—just an establishment's way to please the customer. Although big sizes seem like great deals, you can easily consume hundreds more calories.

Opting for the medium or small portions may save you a few dollars and tons of calories per month.

The normal serving size of beef, fish, pork, and poultry is oversized in typical restaurants. The typical serving size of all meats should be the size of a deck of cards or about four ounces. Of course this may not fill you up, but it is not the only food that you should eat; add fruits and vegetables to make your meal complete.

Food	One Serving Size
Meat	3 ounces or deck of cards
Rice or pasta	½ cup cooked
Fruit	½ cup
Vegetables (raw)	1 cup
Vegetables (cooked)	½ cup
Soda or juice	8 ounces

Eating smaller portions is extremely important to weight loss. This was proven when one group of people ate a 2,000 calorie meal in one sitting and another group of people ate the same 2,000 calorie meal spaced over an entire day. The study showed when excess calories are consumed at one meal, the body uses what it needs and stores the rest as fat. However, when smaller meals are eaten throughout the day, the body is better able to digest the food, which decreases the likelihood of food being stored as fat. Although quite filling, eating a 2,000 calorie meal may not stop you from wanting to eat more later.

To avoid overeating, order the lunch or smaller portion. Ordering smaller portions may help to reduce calories. The child's portion allows you to enjoy a smaller portion with fewer calories, sometimes at a fraction of the cost. However, the child's portion isn't always the better option; the selections on children's menu are limited and generally less healthy than the assortment available on the main menu.

Perhaps Chez La La doesn't even offer a reduced portions. What now? Halve it or ask for a to-go bag right when ordering your meal. By halving your meal you saved yourself hundreds of unwanted calories, not to mention money. And guess what you have? A meal for later.

Cooking

While making improvements and modifying your diet, you may find that in order to do something right, you just have to do it yourself. There are some benefits to cooking your own food. You know the chef personally; the chef is willing to add the little extras you like; you know if the chef's hands are clean; you know there are no teenagers in back adding their own special ingredients (wink, wink); you know how fresh the food is; the list could go on and on.

Cooking style greatly affects the fat and caloric content. Cooking liquefies and releases some of the fat contained in meat, which also reduces calories. When cooking, it is beneficial to bake, boil, broil, grill, or roast, this allows some of the fat to drip away from the meat. Nonstick cookware cooks food nicely without butters and oils. Carefully cook and wash non-stick cookware, it may scratch easily and slowly release the surface coating into your food, which may be toxic.

Eating Out

"More die in the United States of too much food than of too little."
— John Kenneth Galbraith, The Affluent Society

The food industry spends more than 33 billion dollars per year to push products and hopefully tempt your taste buds to buy its product du jour. And the food industry's strategy is working; it is estimated that 64% of meals are consumed outside of the house. More money is spent on food than numerous recreational activities combined.

Most restaurants are only doing what the general public wants, which is provide the biggest portion of the tastiest food at a reasonable price. This is the restaurants' way of being competitive, making a profit, and surviving through economic turbulence. So, do we blame them?

Losing weight is important, but it must fit in with your lifestyle. Just because you are getting healthy doesn't mean that you have to stop going to restaurants. Some restaurants are cognizant that people want to improve their health and they provide healthy alternatives to the regular menu items. Restaurants aren't required to display nutrition facts, unless they make a claim that a menu item is healthy. Restaurants may not want to advertise that certain meals have over 2,500 calories that would ruin your 1,500 calorie dessert. So you may have to put forth some effort to find the information you seek. Some restaurants provide nutrition information online or upon request, which can help you make informed dietary decisions. However, be careful; even if the information is available it may not be completely accurate. As a knowledgeable food consumer, it is important to be able to evaluate the nutritional value of your imminent meal.

There are a couple of things that you can do to help maximize your efforts while dining out. Watch out for the fried and fatty appetizers; the free accouterments like bread, chips, crackers, and dips; the fatty dressings and extras that accompany salads; the serving size of the main dish; the extra sides and condiments that accompany the meal; and the oh so tasty desserts.

But maybe the restaurant hasn't yet considered health conscious individuals, but that is still not a reason for you to interrupt your plans. Do not be afraid to ask questions at the restaurant. Talk to the waiter to see what substitutions and alterations can be made. It is important to know as much as possible about the food you eat, especially if it can negatively impact your health and undo your progress. Who knows, with enough inquiries and requests the restaurant may see the value in offering healthier options on the menu. Seek and you shall find better options.

There are so many ways to make food healthy; it's just like having your cake and eating it too. Instead of fries, order fruit or a salad. Instead of a steak, order a salad with a petite steak; you only need a couple of ounces of meat anyway.

While dining at restaurants, the ingredients and preparation of foods may affect your decision of what to eat. Some of the options that may be available include:

Fatty fixins	Descriptions
Alfredo	Cream
Au beurre	With butter
Au gratin	With cheese
Basted	Sauce
Bathed	Sauce
Battered	Coated
Bérnaise	Egg yolks and butter
Bechamel	Heavy cream, flour, and butter
Breaded	Coated
Buttery	Dairy
Coated	Breaded
Creamy	Dairy
Crispy	Fried in oil
Deep fried	Fried in oil
Dipped	Sauce
Fritter	Fried
Fritto	Fried
Gravy	Meat drippings & flour
Hollandaise	Butter and egg yolk
Marinated	Sauce
Oil	100% liquid fat
Pan-fried	Oil
Rich	With butter or oil
Sautéed	With butter or oil
Tempura	Battered and fried

Buffets, glorious little island stands filled with food, offer all you can eat until you need to be transported out by hand truck. Buffets don't have to be bad. Put on your food evaluator hat. First, search for the healthier items like fruits, vegetables, and salads and then save a little room for a sample of the other appetizing fare.

You gotta love fast food. It's tasty, fast, and cheap, but is generally heavily refined and fattening. Americans can't get enough of it; in 2001 we spent more than 110 billion dollars dining at fast food restaurants. Daily, almost 25% of Americans dine at fast food restaurants for at least one meal. Before, during, or after a hectic day, fast food may seem like a good solution to hunger. But most fast food doesn't supply your body the nutrients that it needs to do its best work. If you want your body to shed extra pounds, it's going to need the proper nutrients; don't just feed it any garbage that you pick up from the side of the road.

Aside from toppings like lettuce and tomatoes, fast food is generally canned, dehydrated, freeze-dried, frozen, prepackaged, and severely lacking in nutritional value. Most of it is light on fiber while heavy on the calories and fat, but it does not have to be all bad.

Make fast food work for you. Say "no" to the condiments and sauces. Considering most fast food is fattening already, it shouldn't need to hide behind calorie-intense condiments. When ordering fast food, tell them to veggie it up with extra vegetables like tomatoes and lettuce. Eliminate the dairy; tell them to cut cheese—in a good way. Eat sandwiches and burgers open-faced with one slice of bread. Most bread at fast food restaurants is refined and nutrient void, it may help fill up your tummy and fanny, but that is it. To get full, there are better options, so save the calories for better foods. By doing so, you can have your fast food and a healthy body too!

While a soda pop goes great with fast food, drinks are an excellent place to save some calories. In lieu of ordering a soda, have a water. You will not only save calories, but money too. The calories and the money may not seem significant on one visit; however, over a year the savings can be pretty substantial to your pocket and waistline, depending on how much and how many times you skipped the soda.

There are many things that just go hand in hand like cake and icing and salad and dressing, but that doesn't mean that there is not room for improvement. The same goes for fast food and French fries. French fries are a tasty accompaniment to fast foods; however, they are scorched in oil, dusted with salt, and full of empty calories. While French fries may be fine every so often, it is much better to select healthier foods. In lieu of French fries, add vegetables, fruits, or whole grains.

If you plan to dine at a fast food establishment, you can always order your main dish while supplying your own side. This is the best of both worlds; eating what you like while still giving your body the nutrients that it needs.

A recent study revealed a significant discrepancy between the calories reported on nutrition labels versus the actual calorie content of restaurant entrees and grocery store frozen food entrees. The study showed there is an average of 18% more calories in commercially prepared food versus what is actually reported on the label. However, some restaurant meals actually had twice as many calories as reported. The grocery store frozen food items had an average of 8% more calories. One factor that may contribute to the significant discrepancy between actual and reported calories of commercially prepared food is failing to include the calories of the side dishes. Some side dishes actually pack calories comparable to the main dish.

Dieters solely relying on nutrition labels may be in jeopardy of gaining at least 10 pounds per year. Although it is a good practice to review nutrition labels, it should not be your only line of defense. Losing weight is a battle that is won through knowledge, exercise, and perseverance.

Keep a Journal

Food journals or diaries can be an important factor to successful dieting. We are not a one-size-fits-all world. What work for someone or even everyone else, may not work for you. You need to know what works for you and a food journal is the perfect way to learn this information. From your journal entries you may find out why you have plateaued, what foods help you lose weight faster, what foods slow your progress, and how different activities affect your weight loss. Food journals can assist in monitoring the amount of weight that you have gained or lost because the information is specific and accurate to you.

Monitoring your meals can make a world of difference to your progress. Each meal can be a learning experience. Before you eat, stop and evaluate the meal. Is it nutritious? Will it help provide your body with nutrients? Will you feel guilty about eating it later? How does the food make you feel? Monitor and record when, where, why, what, and how you feel before and after you eat. Analyzing your actions and feelings will help you better understand your eating and help you make changes. This will require you to be in tune with your body. Some signs of discomfort or intolerance may be very subtle, hardly recognizable, but if you carefully monitor your body and feelings you may learn new information that will facilitate improvements in your weight and health.

In your journal, include every single item that you eat, even if it is as small as a Hershey's Kiss. It is important that you are brutally honest; besides, you are the only one who has to see it. Your honesty and good recording skills will help you analyze how your diet affects you, including what you do right and what needs adjustment.

Without an accurate assessment and careful reflection, it is difficult to determine how various foods impact the way you feel and the rate you lose weight. The analysis of an accurate and detailed food journal can provide a wealth of information that may lead to improvements.

Journaling also can be very therapeutic. A lot can happen during the day that can overwhelm and depress the mood, and it may be beneficial to reflect over daily events. Journaling allows time for observance, reflection, and meditation of different events that took place during the day. Failure to resolve daily issues may impede your body's ability to properly resolve issues and create additional stress.

Children

"Children have never been very good at listening to their elders, but they have never failed to imitate them."
— JAMES BALDWIN (1924-1987).
NOBODY KNOWS MY NAME: MORE NOTES
OF A NATIVE SON, 3, 1961.

Children, like adults, experience issues with food, weight, and health. Children's diets are especially important because many of them are starting to experience the same diseases that affect obese adults, which can be serious and even deadly. That is why it is crucial to provide children with guidance and knowledge that will promote good eating habits for a lifetime. Autopsies of many children who were killed in accidents revealed the beginning stages of heart disease due to poor diets. Research studies reveal that being overweight while young is more dangerous than in adulthood. More often than not, overweight children become overweight adults. According to the *Journal of Pediatrics* two million adolescents aged 12–19 are considered pre-diabetic.

They are cute and cuddly, and sometimes it is very hard to tell them "no," especially when they say that they are hungry or need a snack; however, it is also important to avoid overindulging children with food, candy, and sugary beverages. After children have had a reasonable sized meal or a snack, and their hunger still persists, they should be offered fruits, vegetables, and water to help appease their appetite.

When implementing a better diet for yourself, it is important to do the same thing for your children. Eating habits become engrained in children and can last a lifetime. Establishing good eating habits and routines is one of the most important lessons that you can teach your children. You are a role model for them. Studies have shown that eating habits can have a more significant effect on weight and health than genetics.

While changing children's food regimen:
+ Emphasize water
+ Blend frozen fruits
+ Gradually eliminate sodas and fruit juice
+ Let children select fruit at the grocery store
+ Lead by example—eat fresh fruits and vegetables

Although you may think that children are too young to understand healthy eating strategies, they might just surprise you. Take the time to explain the benefits and detriments of various foods. This will empower kids and help them make good decisions, even when you are not around. Who better to keep you honest and on the straight and narrow, but your kids? As soon as you veer off the road of healthiness, they will surely remind you of everything that you have taught them.

Some children may be resistant to a change in their diet, but as the parent, it is your responsibility to make improvements to their health and broaden their appreciation for different foods that they will grow to enjoy and love. Have you ever heard a song and didn't like it? But after hearing it over and over you were like, "It's actually not that bad!" Same thing with foods, you have to give them a chance; maybe it was the way that they were prepared, a seasoning, or a sauce. Nonetheless, don't cheat your kids out of good nutrients. While children may not instantly like new fruits and vegetables, it is important that they get the opportunity to try them. Give your kids multiple opportunities to appreciate new foods. Seeing you regularly enjoy fruits and vegetables may pique their interest.

With today's busy lifestyles, many children are eating more of their meals outside of the home. Many of the food choices available away from the home lack the nutritional value that children need to maintain good health and weight. Providing children a breakfast and lunch from home can ensure that they are receiving the important nutrients needed.

The food industry spends billions a year on multimedia advertising to capture the public's interest. Children are very impressionable; while this type of targeted approach is acceptable in the US, other countries like Ireland, Norway, and Sweden have taken proactive steps to eliminate the allure of advertisers to children. Make sure your influence is stronger than the marketers and your kids are receiving the right message about food.

Reward

"There are no shortcuts to any place worth going."
— BEVERLY SILLS

Losing weight is a tremendous reward, but it doesn't stop there. Improving the way that you eat may generate additional benefits to your body like a reduction in acne, fatigue, sleep disorders, and health complications. There is a lot to win, so stick with it and put your best effort forth. Reaffirm daily why you are modifying your diet; make a list of the positive rewards that you will reap by losing weight. Thank your body, not with sugary and sweet rewards, but with food that will actually nourish and revitalize it. Additional rewards include, but are not limited to: more energy, better health, and a sense of accomplishment.

Conclusion

Losing weight is not only about what you what; it is about your overall approach to food and how it impacts your diets and health. By planning and making thoughtful dietary decisions you will be one step closer to reaching your weight loss goals.

Maximizing Life 11

ATING HEALTHY IS IMPORTANT, but living healthy is equally important; they go hand in hand, and if you are only doing one or the other, you may not get the results you are looking for. To reap the biggest payoff, go all the way.

Sunlight is an important part of vitamin D absorption. The body is able to manufacture vitamin D with exposure to sunshine. As little as fifteen minutes of direct sunlight per day can help strengthen bones. Skin color affects the body's ability to absorb sunlight and manufacture vitamin D. Dark skin essentially functions as sunblock, and more time may be needed to absorb sufficient sunlight. The lighter the skin, the easier sunlight is absorbed and care should be taken to avoid overexposure and burning.

Sleep

Sleep does a body good, so good in fact, lack of sleep promotes diabetes, high blood pressure, and memory loss. Without proper rest, individuals are more likely to be energy-deprived. When energy-deprived, many people tend to overeat in an attempt to increase their energy level, which may negatively impact attempts to improve health and lose weight.

Lack of sleep disturbs the hormone levels within the body. Studies show that people who get five or less hours of sleep per night have increased levels of ghrelin, a hormone that stimulates appetite, perhaps to compensate for the lack of energy due to sleep deprivation. Lack of sleep hampers the body's ability to function properly. Research has proven that individuals who get adequate amounts of rest are healthier.

Researchers also believe that sleep supports the development of growth hormones, without which the body is more likely to develop additional fat tissue and less muscle. Essentially, seven to eight hours of sleep is required to reenergize the body, harness the fat-burning effects of the growth hormone, and reduce cortisol levels.

Sixty-nine percent of Americans report having a sleep disturbance that impairs their ability to gain a good night's rest; this fact may contribute to the obesity equation. To improve sleep, the following tips are recommended:

+ Avoid alcohol
+ Keep the sleeping area cool: 63°–70° F
+ Refrain from taking a nap after 4:00 p.m.
+ Establish a routine sleep and wake schedule
+ Take a warm bath one to two hours before bedtime
+ Relax mentally: read or watch TV—whatever works
+ Do not exercise at least two hours before your go to sleep
+ Stop eating at least two to three hours before you go to sleep
+ Use a floor fan or a sound machine to drown out random noises

Eliminate Negatives
Stress

With the hustle and bustle of life, it is difficult to incorporate everything. Some things may fall by the wayside, but your health should be a non-negotiable. Making your health a priority and taking care of yourself must be first on your list. Although taking care of yourself may seem selfish, it is necessary. You have to take care of yourself first, to adequately take care of everything and everyone else. Taking care of yourself means having to say "no." People who are unwilling to say "no" place a considerable amount of stress on themselves, which is injurious to good health. Wellness comes from being in control and able to properly manage obligations.

Managing stress is important to your health, but it is also important to your weight loss efforts. Lack of sleep, as well as stress, increases cortisol levels. High cortisol levels have an adverse effect on the body and may cause the following complications:

+ Osteoporosis
+ Fluid retention
+ Muscle weakness
+ High blood pressure
+ Elevated blood sugar
+ Diminished memory
+ Increased food consumption

Many people are mal-equipped to handle stress and immediately turn to food to help them temporarily feel better during troubles; however, this is not a permanent solution, it does not solve any problem and may further deteriorate health. During childhood, stressful situations are often soothed with treats like candy or ice cream. It is no wonder why as adults, many of us return to familiar foods to get soothing comfort. It is important to be prepared for the body's desire to eat comforting foods; however, more suitable foods should be available while enduring stress such as fruits and vegetables.

Some stress may be energizing; however, consistently putting yourself into stressful situations may diminish health and promote weight gain. Find a way to deal with everyday issues that are not associated with food like acknowledging problems, talking about problems with others, and creating good resolutions. Deal with problems by outwardly expressing concerns, rather than bottling up the issues inside. It may be useful to employ some de-stressing techniques to help alleviate stress. Some additional ways to reduce stress include:

+ Walking
+ Cooking
+ Reading
+ A massage
+ Meditating
+ A warm bath
+ Enjoying nature
+ Soaking your feet
+ Listening to music

Find your passion. If you know what it is, great! If not, then experiment with different activities that pique your interest. When participating in an activity that you love, time passes effortlessly, alleviating the need to fill time with needless food and fodder.

Smoking

"One thousand Americans stop smoking every day—by dying."
— Unknown

Everyone knows that smoking is bad for your health so we'll skip that part, but did you know that it makes you fat and old? Many people profess that it keeps the weight off because they do not eat as much when their hands and mouth are busy. If you're worried about your hands and mouth, get a piece of gum and a gaming device. The truth is smoking doesn't keep the weight off, but it actually keeps the weight on. Smoking and drinking promote fat storage in the stomach area. Your body needs a continual supply of oxygen for cellular activity,

ny people *initially* love, or even like exercise, but it is
mproving health. You may even get to the place that it
r you, next you may like, and eventually you may find
live without it. Exercise may enhance the way that you
. Once you make exercise part of your life, it should be
ntain. Studies show that it takes approximately three
blish a routine.

rds of exercise can last throughout the day. In addition,
des a mountain of benefits, including:

ss

ep

ergy

etite

scle

y fat

estion

sique

munity

-image

ulation

abolism

ar levels

weight

f cancer

arthritis

ity of life

d pressure

+ Improve toxin removal

+ Improve calcium absorption

+ Increase level of endorphins

+ Increase in strength and
stamina

+ Reduce the risk of type 2
diabetes

+ Help decrease depression and
improve mood

+ Reduce abominable
abdominal fat

+ Reduce the risk for obesity
related diseases

+ Help prevent impotence

+ Help prevent osteoporosis

+ Improve cardiac and
pulmonary functions

rcise, fat dominates the body and muscles fade away,
d less food for you to gain more and more weight.
ur body without being forced to do so. Make your

otherwise known as metabolism. When you smoke, your body has
limited resources to do work, so the body's functioning is limited
and your metabolism is slowed. Smoking deprives cells of oxygen
and increases the amount of damaging free radicals in the body. In
addition to reducing the oxygen in the body, smoking increases the
body's exposure to nicotine, an addictive irritant.

If you smoke, quitting may be one of the hardest things that you
will ever do, but you can do it. In time, quitting will get easier and
you will be grateful to yourself for kicking the habit. There are also
a lot of tools available to help you stop smoking like the patch, pill,
and therapy. Pick the tool that is right for you and get on the road to
recovery and improved health.

Plateau

*"The older you get, the tougher it is to lose weight because by
then, your body and your fat are really good friends."*
— UNKNOWN

There are many reasons why weight loss plateaus. Plateaus may be
attributed to activity level, age, allergies, body composition, calorie
consumption, food, food sensitivities, metabolic rate, set points, and
weight. The good news is that you can analyze what is going on with
your body to rev up your weight loss. Generally weight loss efforts
improve with additional effort.

As we grow older it is more difficult to lose weight because the
metabolism slows with age. Weight may float away in your teens and
twenties without much effort, but this may not be true after thirty.
To get better results, you have to do more.

As you lose weight your body will require fewer calories, so it
may be harder to lose additional weight and losing the last pounds
may be the hardest; however, you can combat this dilemma. Body
fat keeps the metabolism in low gear. To increase the metabolism

and burn additional calories increase muscle mass. Muscle burns more calories than fat and can help you lose weight, even by doing nothing at all.

Set points can stall weight loss. A set point is the weight the body maintains naturally. Don't worry if your goal is to lose more weight. It can still be achieved, but it is going to take more effort. Also, consider that everybody is different and not meant to be a size 00, 0, or even a 6. Settle on a healthy weight that you can comfortably maintain without driving yourself bonkers.

Many different factors determine your body's energy requirement. When your body's energy requirement has been met, anything extra consumed may be stored as fat. It doesn't take much to add major pounds per year; by consuming just 66 extra calories per day you'll gain one pound per month, 12 pounds per year, and 120 pounds per decade! Yawzaa!

Reducing or eliminating foods that cause allergic reactions may promote weight loss. The foods that cause the most allergic reaction include eggs, fish, milk, peanuts, shellfish, soy, tree nuts, and wheat. Allergic reactions within the body promote inflammation and impede the body's ability to function optimally. But when you reduce or eliminate foods that trigger an inflammatory response, the body may be better able to manage digestion and produce weight loss. If food creates a negative reaction, the body will be busy trying to heal and neutralize the problems. Eliminate all foods that your body does not tolerate, is sensitive to, or promotes any other negative reaction. Select foods that are going to amplify, not squander, your efforts.

Reviewing your food journal can provide a lot of insightful information about your weight loss. If you hit a plateau you can review your journal for a time when your efforts were more successful. This information is specific to you and may help you make improvements.

Illuminate the Positives
Exercise

*If you have not exercise
physician to see if there
with you exercising. Alth
get the pounds off, st

*The only exercise some people ge
down their friends, side-stepping
— U

Approximately 78% of Ame
physical and outdoor activity.
and well-being. Lack of physic
to obesity. The body needs ade
sumption, facilitate weight los

While eating well is part
for exercise and what it does
work together synergistically
the weight off. Exercising ma
anything new there is an adj

Although there are clai
exercise, you can, if you like
to slow your metabolism do
to eat, you'll pack on the po
when you lose weight, you
gain weight it is generally

So you know that you
reasons bouncing around
While you're debating wi
read on to find some rebutt

Not ma
essential to
doesn't both
that you can
look and fee
easier to ma
weeks to esta

The rewa
exercise prov

+ Reduce str
+ Improve sl
+ Increase en
+ Reduce app
+ Increase m
+ Reduce bod
+ Improve dig
+ Improve ph
+ Enhance im
+ Improve sel
+ Improve cir
+ Increase me
+ Improve sug
+ Help manag
+ Reduce risk
+ Help preven
+ Improve qua
+ Improve blo

Without exe
requiring less a
Fat can't leave y

fat uncomfortable and slowly but surely it will leave. Without the effort, it's just too comfortable and receiving all of the nourishment needed to stay put.

Just like age, weight is only a number, especially if you exercise regularly. Exercising regularly builds muscle and it weighs more than fat; therefore, your weight loss may stall, but you may see the results in your physique and even in smaller clothes sizes. Exercise prevents muscle atrophy, which reduces the development of fat. Exercise builds muscle that burns as much as five times or an additional 70 calories per hour more than regular body tissue; that alone is reason to exercise.

As early as the mid-thirties, both men and women start to lose bone density; however, regular exercise can reduce and even reverse the reduction of bone density. In addition, exercise promotes the development of several neurotransmitters such as dopamine, norepinephrine, and serotonin that positively affect the body for several hours.

"A journey of a thousand miles must begin with a single step."
— CHINESE PROVERB

Even if you're not ready to begin an official exercise routine, just do something. Any increased movement will increase your metabolism. Whether wiggling, jiggling, dancing, walking, cycling, cleaning, or swimming, whatever gets your blood pumping—it all counts. Anything more than you are currently doing is a great start. Movement facilitates weight loss endeavors and the more weight you lose, the easier it will be to enjoy more activities. Some great ways to increase daily activity include, but are not limited to:

+ Shop daily
+ Do yard work
+ Take the stairs
+ Clean the house

- Cook versus take-out
- Stand in lieu of sitting
- Play outdoors with your kids
- Park further from the entrance
- Walk or bicycle instead of driving
- Walk the whole mall or grocery store

"You may delay, but time will not."
— BENJAMIN FRANKLIN

Don't let procrastination rob you of your health. Procrastination is a nasty little bug and it often flares up when exercise comes into the picture. All kinds of important appointments, errands, and events materialize right of out thin air to delay what really needs to start today. There are so many reasons not to exercise: too busy, too tired, not ready, too hard, too inconvenient. Start exercising against all odds, even if it is not the grand exercise routine that you'd idealistically like to implement. Starting today gets you a day closer to your goal, and time is too precious to waste. Studies show that even modest exercise can provide benefits.

If left to chance, exercise may not happen and you're only cheating yourself. You may think that there is just not enough time in your day to add an exercise regimen, but that is not true. The truth is if you really wanted to do it, you would find a way to incorporate it into your day. Make exercise a non-negotiable, scheduled part of your day. Instead of trying to figure out when you are going to fit in exercise, put exercise in first and determine how you are going to fit in everything else. Besides, almost everything else is replaceable—errands, homes, jobs—but life is not replaceable.

"Discipline is the bridge between goals and accomplishments."
— JIM ROHN

Workouts can be planted at any point throughout the day. You never know what you can do until you try, so it's time to put in some effort. Just start. There are many types of exercises; you just have to find the ones that you like and that fit in with your lifestyle. Experiment with a couple of different exercises and times until you find the right one for you. The important thing is to keep searching for the right fit.

Some of the alternatives you can try are:

+ Work out after work
+ Work out during lunch
+ Wake up a little earlier to exercise

Don't wear yourself out and thereby make exercise a horrible experience that you'd never want to repeat again. Exercise does not have to be intense or painful to be effective. In fact, strenuous exercise can be more detrimental than beneficial. Strenuous exercise can be defined as intense exercise exceeding two hours per day. For women, too much exercise can cease menstruation and escalate the aging process.

If you haven't exercised in a long time, start small, even little efforts can be beneficial. Exercise doesn't have to be very time consuming. You can start off with just a few minutes a day and work your way up to the recommended 30 minutes. Exercise can be broken up into pieces throughout the day. For instance three 10-minute walks throughout the day count as 30 minutes of exercise; however, this should not be confused with regular walking. Exercise at least three days per week, more if possible. Research shows that low to moderate exercise three to four times per week, is more beneficial than intense exercise.

Going to the gym can be an intimidating adventure. Moseying into a building full of fit folks getting more fit may be unnerving; it may feel as though every eyeball is piercing your skin and you may wonder—what am I doing here? Fortunately, only your world revolves around you. Most people at the gym are just like you—thinking about themselves. Even if they are thinking about you, forget about 'em, you've got work to do.

> *"The difference between the impossible and the*
> *possible lies in a person's determination."*
> — TOMMY LASORDA

So you're not concerned about the gym gurus anymore, but now the problem du jour is your lack of energy—you couldn't possibly go to the gym. Besides, there are so many things to do. Going to the gym is a luxury that only stay-at-home moms and muscle bound maniacs can indulge in. NOT! You're an adult: set a schedule, prioritize, and commit. Bigger people before have done it and bigger people after you will do it too. The question now is, will you? How committed are you? How much do you want it? What are you willing to do to make it happen?

I don't have enough money to work out. Great! That cuts out a lot of complications and pondering about that equipment, clothes, shoes, or gyms to join. No money means you're walking. Walking at a brisk pace is a great form of exercise that can be done virtually anywhere—no equipment necessary. Brisk walking burns up to 70% more calories than sitting around.

Even if you don't like walking, there are still a variety of exercises that don't require extra equipment like calisthenics, which uses a series of different movements to enhance the body's strength and flexibility. Different calisthenics exercises include: crunches, dips, jumping jacks, leg lifts, lunges, push-ups, sit-ups, and squats.

I don't really want to exercise; I'll just cut back and diet more. Nuh uhh! Not going to work. Exercising intensifies the effort of dieting; you'll get improvements faster and maintain them longer. At first exercising may feel like a chore, but it may get easier with time if you continue to exercise on a regular basis.

I would work out, but I'm not physically able to. It is important to accurately assess your abilities. Exercise that is physically uncomfortable is not the same as being physically unable. If you truly can't exercise then you have a free pass. Just joking. There are sedentary or bed exercises that you can do. Don't discount the value of these exercises; they will get you closer to your goal. While sitting in a chair or lying down in the bed, you can do leg and arm lifts. Lift your body part up and then move it back and forth or in a circular motion. This is great exercise, and if you don't believe it, try it; you will feel the burn shortly. To intensify any workout, add a couple of pounds of weights. No need to overdo it, a pound or two is enough to strengthen muscle. If you're worried that the added weight will have you looking like the hulk, don't. It will just help build muscle to reduce fat and burn calories.

I don't care; I will never exercise outside of my house. OK. You're the boss, but don't let that stop you from exercising. There is a variety of exercise equipment that can be purchased economically for the home, from videos, to exercise balls, to exercise machines, to quality gym equipment. A quick trip to your local sports store or a search on the internet will put you into contact with everything that you need to transform your home into an exercise oasis.

Exercising with a partner can be great and make the time fly by. However, it is essential that both partners share a commitment to exercise; if not, it may reduce the level of motivation for one of the partners. If exercise plans fall through, don't let your partner's schedule spoil your workout. Your partner's absence does not mean that you have a free pass. Have an alternative exercise plan or partner. If your partner doesn't work, remember coordinating exercise plans for one is easier than coordinating exercise plans for two.

Once you get started, it is important to develop a well-rounded exercise regimen that includes a variety of exercises to help you meet and maintain your weight and health goals. Well-rounded exercise routines include cardiovascular, stretching, and resistance exercises.

Exercise is not an optional part of the equation. Exercise isn't all fun and tickles, it's hard. That's why it's called a workout. Exercise enhances your efforts to lose weight. Any type of exercise is better than none at all, so get moving. Exercise takes effort, time, and commitment; but if you follow through, the results will be more than worth it and you will be proud of your accomplishments. The sooner you get started, the sooner you will reap your rewards. Once you start losing weight it may be the igniter to keep you moving.

Progress

There are many different ideas regarding how and when to check your weight loss progress. Ultimately, the timing is up to you. The different options include a variety of intervals that provide distinct advantages and disadvantages. Checking weight regularly is a practice of many people who have successfully lost weight and kept it off. Daily checks help keep close tabs of what works and what doesn't.

Although daily checks may seem like too much, it is helpful to monitor weight before pounds are securely fastened to your hinny. Excess weight can sneak up on you like a ghost in a graveyard; you don't realize it's there until it scares you. The best way to avoid the fright is to monitor your weight daily. Catch those sneaky, pesky pounds. Monitoring weight gain will allow you to make immediate changes in your diet and exercise routine to keep you on the right path. Weekly checks give a broader overview. Never checking your weight is not for everyone, but may be for people who are making changes to improve health, rather than to lose weight.

When checking your weight, a digital scale may come in handy. Regular scales may not report small weight loss wins; however, a digital scale can provide you with your weight down to the ounce. Knowing that you have lost a couple of ounces may boost your motivation. In addition, some digital scales can even provide you with an analysis of your body fat. Even if you haven't lost any weight, otherwise known as metabolism. When you smoke, your body has limited resources to do work, so the body's functioning is limited and your metabolism is slowed. Smoking deprives cells of oxygen and increases the amount of damaging free radicals in the body. In addition to reducing the oxygen in the body, smoking increases the body's exposure to nicotine, an addictive irritant.

If you smoke, quitting may be one of the hardest things that you will ever do, but you can do it. In time, quitting will get easier and you will be grateful to yourself for kicking the habit. There are also a lot of tools available to help you stop smoking like the patch, pill, and therapy. Pick the tool that is right for you and get on the road to recovery and improved health.

Plateau

> *"The older you get, the tougher it is to lose weight because by then, your body and your fat are really good friends."*
> — Unknown

There are many reasons why weight loss plateaus. Plateaus may be attributed to activity level, age, allergies, body composition, calorie consumption, food, food sensitivities, metabolic rate, set points, and weight. The good news is that you can analyze what is going on with your body to rev up your weight loss. Generally weight loss efforts improve with additional effort.

As we grow older it is more difficult to lose weight because the metabolism slows with age. Weight may float away in your teens and twenties without much effort, but this may not be true after thirty. To get better results, you have to do more.

As you lose weight your body will require fewer calories, so it may be harder to lose additional weight and losing the last pounds may be the hardest; however, you can combat this dilemma. Body fat keeps the metabolism in low gear. To increase the metabolism and burn additional calories increase muscle mass. Muscle burns more calories than fat and can help you lose weight, even by doing nothing at all.

Set points can stall weight loss. A set point is the weight the body maintains naturally. Don't worry if your goal is to lose more weight. It can still be achieved, but it is going to take more effort. Also, consider that everybody is different and not meant to be a size 00, 0, or even a 6. Settle on a healthy weight that you can comfortably maintain without driving yourself bonkers.

Many different factors determine your body's energy requirement. When your body's energy requirement has been met, anything extra consumed may be stored as fat. It doesn't take much to add major pounds per year; by consuming just 66 extra calories per day you'll gain one pound per month, 12 pounds per year, and 120 pounds per decade! Yawzaa!

Reducing or eliminating foods that cause allergic reactions may promote weight loss. The foods that cause the most allergic reaction include eggs, fish, milk, peanuts, shellfish, soy, tree nuts, and wheat. Allergic reactions within the body promote inflammation and impede the body's ability to function optimally. But when you reduce or eliminate foods that trigger an inflammatory response, the body may be better able to manage digestion and produce weight loss. If food creates a negative reaction, the body will be busy trying to heal and neutralize the problems. Eliminate all foods that your body does not tolerate, is sensitive to, or promotes any other negative reaction. Select foods that are going to amplify, not squander, your efforts.

Reviewing your food journal can provide a lot of insightful information about your weight loss. If you hit a plateau you can review your journal for a time when your efforts were more successful. This information is specific to you and may help you make improvements.

Illuminate the Positives
Exercise

*If you have not exercised in a while, consult your
physician to see if there may be any risks associated
with you exercising. Although you may be anxious to
get the pounds off, start slow to avoid injuries.

*The only exercise some people get is jumping to conclusions, running
down their friends, side-stepping responsibility, and pushing their luck!*
— UNKNOWN

Approximately 78% of Americans have sedentary lifestyles, void of
physical and outdoor activity. Physical activity is important to health
and well-being. Lack of physical activity is a significant contributor
to obesity. The body needs adequate exercise to improve calorie consumption, facilitate weight loss, and build muscle.

While eating well is part of the solution, there is no substitute
for exercise and what it does for the body. A good diet and exercise
work together synergistically to help you lose weight faster and keep
the weight off. Exercising may not sound like much fun, but as with
anything new there is an adjustment period.

Although there are claims that you can lose weight without
exercise, you can, if you like starving yourself; but that is only going
to slow your metabolism down more, so when you eventually start
to eat, you'll pack on the pounds like a hibernating bear. Generally
when you lose weight, you lose muscle and a little fat, but when you
gain weight it is generally only fat.

So you know that you have to exercise, but you have millions of
reasons bouncing around in your head of why you just can't do it.
While you're debating with yourself, if you really want to exercise
read on to find some rebuttals and reasons that support you exercising.

Not many people *initially* love, or even like exercise, but it is essential to improving health. You may even get to the place that it doesn't bother you, next you may like, and eventually you may find that you can't live without it. Exercise may enhance the way that you look and feel. Once you make exercise part of your life, it should be easier to maintain. Studies show that it takes approximately three weeks to establish a routine.

The rewards of exercise can last throughout the day. In addition, exercise provides a mountain of benefits, including:

+ Reduce stress
+ Improve sleep
+ Increase energy
+ Reduce appetite
+ Increase muscle
+ Reduce body fat
+ Improve digestion
+ Improve physique
+ Enhance immunity
+ Improve self-image
+ Improve circulation
+ Increase metabolism
+ Improve sugar levels
+ Help manage weight
+ Reduce risk of cancer
+ Help prevent arthritis
+ Improve quality of life
+ Improve blood pressure
+ Improve toxin removal
+ Improve calcium absorption
+ Increase level of endorphins
+ Increase in strength and stamina
+ Reduce the risk of type 2 diabetes
+ Help decrease depression and improve mood
+ Reduce abominable abdominal fat
+ Reduce the risk for obesity related diseases
+ Help prevent impotence
+ Help prevent osteoporosis
+ Improve cardiac and pulmonary functions

Without exercise, fat dominates the body and muscles fade away, requiring less and less food for you to gain more and more weight. Fat can't leave your body without being forced to do so. Make your fat uncomfortable and slowly but surely it will leave. Without the effort, it's just too comfortable and receiving all of the nourishment needed to stay put.

Just like age, weight is only a number, especially if you exercise regularly. Exercising regularly builds muscle and it weighs more than fat; therefore, your weight loss may stall, but you may see the results in your physique and even in smaller clothes sizes. Exercise prevents muscle atrophy, which reduces the development of fat. Exercise builds muscle that burns as much as five times or an additional 70 calories per hour more than regular body tissue; that alone is reason to exercise.

As early as the mid-thirties, both men and women start to lose bone density; however, regular exercise can reduce and even reverse the reduction of bone density. In addition, exercise promotes the development of several neurotransmitters such as dopamine, norepinephrine, and serotonin that positively affect the body for several hours.

"A journey of a thousand miles must begin with a single step."
— CHINESE PROVERB

Even if you're not ready to begin an official exercise routine, just do something. Any increased movement will increase your metabolism. Whether wiggling, jiggling, dancing, walking, cycling, cleaning, or swimming, whatever gets your blood pumping—it all counts. Anything more than you are currently doing is a great start. Movement facilitates weight loss endeavors and the more weight you lose, the easier it will be to enjoy more activities. Some great ways to increase daily activity include, but are not limited to:

+ Shop daily
+ Do yard work
+ Take the stairs
+ Clean the house

+ Cook versus take-out
+ Stand in lieu of sitting
+ Play outdoors with your kids
+ Park further from the entrance
+ Walk or bicycle instead of driving
+ Walk the whole mall or grocery store

"You may delay, but time will not."
— BENJAMIN FRANKLIN

Don't let procrastination rob you of your health. Procrastination is a nasty little bug and it often flares up when exercise comes into the picture. All kinds of important appointments, errands, and events materialize right of out thin air to delay what really needs to start today. There are so many reasons not to exercise: too busy, too tired, not ready, too hard, too inconvenient. Start exercising against all odds, even if it is not the grand exercise routine that you'd idealistically like to implement. Starting today gets you a day closer to your goal, and time is too precious to waste. Studies show that even modest exercise can provide benefits.

If left to chance, exercise may not happen and you're only cheating yourself. You may think that there is just not enough time in your day to add an exercise regimen, but that is not true. The truth is if you really wanted to do it, you would find a way to incorporate it into your day. Make exercise a non-negotiable, scheduled part of your day. Instead of trying to figure out when you are going to fit in exercise, put exercise in first and determine how you are going to fit in everything else. Besides, almost everything else is replaceable—errands, homes, jobs—but life is not replaceable.

"Discipline is the bridge between goals and accomplishments."
— JIM ROHN

Workouts can be planted at any point throughout the day. You never know what you can do until you try, so it's time to put in some effort. Just start. There are many types of exercises; you just have to find the ones that you like and that fit in with your lifestyle. Experiment with a couple of different exercises and times until you find the right one for you. The important thing is to keep searching for the right fit.

Some of the alternatives you can try are:
+ Work out after work
+ Work out during lunch
+ Wake up a little earlier to exercise

Don't wear yourself out and thereby make exercise a horrible experience that you'd never want to repeat again. Exercise does not have to be intense or painful to be effective. In fact, strenuous exercise can be more detrimental than beneficial. Strenuous exercise can be defined as intense exercise exceeding two hours per day. For women, too much exercise can cease menstruation and escalate the aging process.

If you haven't exercised in a long time, start small, even little efforts can be beneficial. Exercise doesn't have to be very time consuming. You can start off with just a few minutes a day and work your way up to the recommended 30 minutes. Exercise can be broken up into pieces throughout the day. For instance three 10-minute walks throughout the day count as 30 minutes of exercise; however, this should not be confused with regular walking. Exercise at least three days per week, more if possible. Research shows that low to moderate exercise three to four times per week, is more beneficial than intense exercise.

Going to the gym can be an intimidating adventure. Moseying into a building full of fit folks getting more fit may be unnerving; it may feel as though every eyeball is piercing your skin and you may wonder—what am I doing here? Fortunately, only your world revolves around you. Most people at the gym are just like you—thinking about themselves. Even if they are thinking about you, forget about 'em, you've got work to do.

> *"The difference between the impossible and the*
> *possible lies in a person's determination."*
> — TOMMY LASORDA

So you're not concerned about the gym gurus anymore, but now the problem du jour is your lack of energy—you couldn't possibly go to the gym. Besides, there are so many things to do. Going to the gym is a luxury that only stay-at-home moms and muscle bound maniacs can indulge in. NOT! You're an adult: set a schedule, prioritize, and commit. Bigger people before have done it and bigger people after you will do it too. The question now is, will you? How committed are you? How much do you want it? What are you willing to do to make it happen?

I don't have enough money to work out. Great! That cuts out a lot of complications and pondering about that equipment, clothes, shoes, or gyms to join. No money means you're walking. Walking at a brisk pace is a great form of exercise that can be done virtually anywhere—no equipment necessary. Brisk walking burns up to 70% more calories than sitting around.

Even if you don't like walking, there are still a variety of exercises that don't require extra equipment like calisthenics, which uses a series of different movements to enhance the body's strength and flexibility. Different calisthenics exercises include: crunches, dips, jumping jacks, leg lifts, lunges, push-ups, sit-ups, and squats.

I don't really want to exercise; I'll just cut back and diet more. Nuh uhh! Not going to work. Exercising intensifies the effort of dieting; you'll get improvements faster and maintain them longer. At first exercising may feel like a chore, but it may get easier with time if you continue to exercise on a regular basis.

I would work out, but I'm not physically able to. It is important to accurately assess your abilities. Exercise that is physically uncomfortable is not the same as being physically unable. If you truly can't exercise then you have a free pass. Just joking. There are sedentary or bed exercises that you can do. Don't discount the value of these exercises; they will get you closer to your goal. While sitting in a chair or lying down in the bed, you can do leg and arm lifts. Lift your body part up and then move it back and forth or in a circular motion. This is great exercise, and if you don't believe it, try it; you will feel the burn shortly. To intensify any workout, add a couple of pounds of weights. No need to overdo it, a pound or two is enough to strengthen muscle. If you're worried that the added weight will have you looking like the hulk, don't. It will just help build muscle to reduce fat and burn calories.

I don't care; I will never exercise outside of my house. OK. You're the boss, but don't let that stop you from exercising. There is a variety of exercise equipment that can be purchased economically for the home, from videos, to exercise balls, to exercise machines, to quality gym equipment. A quick trip to your local sports store or a search on the internet will put you into contact with everything that you need to transform your home into an exercise oasis.

Exercising with a partner can be great and make the time fly by. However, it is essential that both partners share a commitment to exercise; if not, it may reduce the level of motivation for one of the partners. If exercise plans fall through, don't let your partner's schedule spoil your workout. Your partner's absence does not mean that you have a free pass. Have an alternative exercise plan or partner. If your partner doesn't work, remember coordinating exercise plans for one is easier than coordinating exercise plans for two.

Once you get started, it is important to develop a well-rounded exercise regimen that includes a variety of exercises to help you meet and maintain your weight and health goals. Well-rounded exercise routines include cardiovascular, stretching, and resistance exercises.

Exercise is not an optional part of the equation. Exercise isn't all fun and tickles, it's hard. That's why it's called a workout. Exercise enhances your efforts to lose weight. Any type of exercise is better than none at all, so get moving. Exercise takes effort, time, and commitment; but if you follow through, the results will be more than worth it and you will be proud of your accomplishments. The sooner you get started, the sooner you will reap your rewards. Once you start losing weight it may be the igniter to keep you moving.

Progress

There are many different ideas regarding how and when to check your weight loss progress. Ultimately, the timing is up to you. The different options include a variety of intervals that provide distinct advantages and disadvantages. Checking weight regularly is a practice of many people who have successfully lost weight and kept it off. Daily checks help keep close tabs of what works and what doesn't.

Although daily checks may seem like too much, it is helpful to monitor weight before pounds are securely fastened to your hinny. Excess weight can sneak up on you like a ghost in a graveyard; you don't realize it's there until it scares you. The best way to avoid the fright is to monitor your weight daily. Catch those sneaky, pesky pounds. Monitoring weight gain will allow you to make immediate changes in your diet and exercise routine to keep you on the right path. Weekly checks give a broader overview. Never checking your weight is not for everyone, but may be for people who are making changes to improve health, rather than to lose weight.

When checking your weight, a digital scale may come in handy. Regular scales may not report small weight loss wins; however, a digital scale can provide you with your weight down to the ounce. Knowing that you have lost a couple of ounces may boost your motivation. In addition, some digital scales can even provide you with an analysis of your body fat. Even if you haven't lost any weight, it may be wonderful to know that you have reduced body fat and increased your muscle mass.

Although weight is important, it should not be the only factor to judge the success of your efforts because that can be very deceiving and discouraging. Success may be camouflaged by muscle weight, which weighs more than fat. If you participate in physical activity, it may increase your muscle mass and there is a good chance that you may maintain or increase your weight. If you experience weight gain or a plateau due to increased muscle mass, it is still a move in the right direction. Don't worry, there are still other ways to confirm your progress.

Weight is not the only important factor in the battle of the bulge; body measurements are important, especially waist circumference. At the beginning of your diet, take measurements at multiple points on your body. After four weeks or another interval of your choice, determine how many inches you have lost. In addition, the tightness or looseness of your clothes can also be a good indicator of how you're progressing.

Changes don't take place overnight. Making improvements to your diet will require time and dedication. Take it one day at a time, put your best effort forth, and you will find success. Reaching your ideal weight would be super fantastic; however, the great news is that a study by the New England Journal of Medicine shows that losing just 10 to 15 percent of your body weight is enough to cause significant health improvements. Remember it is more important to be healthy, than to be thin. Skinny people do not have the monopoly on good health; anyone can take in limited calories while feasting on junk that will eventually muck up good health.

Commitment, Great Expectations, and Goals

*"You must begin to think of yourself as becoming
the person you want to be."*
— David Viscott

Your commitment to improving your diet determines how fast and the extent of the results that you'll achieve. We live in an immediate gratification society. We want everything yesterday, and the same applies to weight loss. As soon as we start a diet, we want to see immediate results that have not developed yet.

Losing weight is hard to do, so much so that the medical community considers maintaining even a 5% weight loss successful because while most dieters may lose weight at one point or another, many of them regrettably regain the weight they have lost and more.

Realistic expectations of weight loss goals should be established before you start your journey. There are some diets that promise insane amounts of weight loss, which may be very hard or nearly impossible to achieve. Expecting to lose 15 pounds per week and only losing one pound can be very frustrating. However, knowing beforehand that losing one pound per week is considered pretty darn good may make a considerable difference. One pound a week does not seem like a lot; however, it is doable, more sustainable, and healthier than losing five pounds per week. And you'll have lost more than 50 pounds in one year!

While superfast weight loss may seem dreamy, it is far from ideal. Dramatic weight loss is most likely the result of water weight loss. In addition, fast weight loss is tough on the body and may cause health complications like gallstones. Diets that promote significant weight loss are generally void of the nutritional content that the body needs.

Losing weight may be a long process, but don't give up. Realize that you didn't put the weight on in one week and it is not going to come off in one week or even a month. If you set unrealistic expectations you may completely abandon your efforts to lose weight. Not seeing immediate results can be discouraging, especially when you work hard; however, if you stick with a good plan you will surely reach your goal, even if the process is slow. Slow and steady wins the race; it's not a cliché for kicks.

Long-term goals can drag on with no end in sight, like working in a deep tunnel, with no light. It is best to have manageable short-term goals. Short-term goals are great because they give direction, inspire, and they're over before you know it. Once you have reached your short-term goal, new goals can be established. When establishing goals it is important to identify the date, duration, goal, menu, and plan.

For example:

Goal	Start	Duration	Menu	Plan
To lose two pounds	January 1st	Two weeks	Eating fruits and vegetables	Exercise 30 minutes 3x per week

We all have that magical number in our heads of the ideal weight. While goals are great, it is important that goals be achievable. Pin thin is not for everyone and may not be the healthiest choice. What good is being skinny if you're riddled with sickness and can't enjoy life? Keep weight goals flexible; instead of narrowing a goal to one particular number, select a range. This will improve chances of success while leaving room to create future goals.

You have to believe that you can reach your goal, even when you slip or hit plateaus, which will happen. Sidetracks and temptations will appear, but your determination to reach your goal must remain strong. Even if you have a setback you must reach inside of yourself and find the motivation to keep going until you achieve success.

"You don't drown by falling in the water.
You drown by staying there."
— UNKNOWN

You may fall off the wagon into a boatload of totally delicious, not even slightly nutritious, delectable goodies. It happens. The important thing to do right after it happens is to deal with it. Get off of your totally satisfied keister and start moving. Take a walk, swim, or clean your house, but don't let that fat make its new home on your butt.

It is easy to slack off and relapse into old comfortable ways, but don't let it happen. When you are tempted to stray, stop, relax, and visualize your goal. See yourself being victorious over your current challenges and reaching your finish line. Visualization is a powerful mental technique that can help you achieve your goals. Dispel any negative thoughts about not achieving your goal. Visualize yourself achieving your goals, step by step, progressively getting closer and closer to your goals. With dedication, motivation, and belief in yourself, you will reach your goals. Think positive. You will do it!

If you don't achieve success in your diet in the first attempt, then you are not alone. The most important thing is your commitment to a healthy lifestyle. If you slip up, don't linger in despair and fall back into bad routines, get back on track as soon as possible.

It is important to remember that nothing and nobody are perfect. This includes you and your diet. Trying to achieve perfection can be disheartening and unsatisfying. Even the smartest and most diligent people have made tons of errors. What separates the successful from the unsuccessful is their ability to keep going, despite failure. You have this ability too. Don't let anything stop you from reaching your goal. Learn from your mistakes and make modifications, but never give up. If you haven't lost weight before, the problem isn't with you, it was with the plan.

Support

Help from others can assist in your weight loss journey. You may benefit from a support group. In support groups you can meet people who have the same issues as you and they may be able to provide you with ideas, motivation, reassurance, support, and tips.

Support groups are not only offered in person, but online as well. There are an abundance of online support groups that get pretty specialized depending on your needs. Sharing experiences in a support group may make your journey a little easier and enjoyable.

Your health lies in your hands. You and only you are responsible for improving your health and crafting the lifestyle that will assist you in being healthy. A support system is good, but you have to put in the effort. Get support for fortification and step up to the challenge.

Eureka!

Eventually you will reach your target weight. After losing weight it is easy to rest of the laurels of your success; however, to keep the prize you have earned it is imperative to be cautious about your daily meals. It is not time to break loose and celebrate with a tub of the cold and creamy, but rather continue with the same plan that got you to the promised land. More important than the time spent losing weight is the time that is spent not losing weight. Maintaining a healthy diet and exercise routine is important to weight maintenance because research studies show that two years after losing weight, nearly 95% of people who have lost 50 pounds or more had regained the weight.

Closing

Every bite is an opportunity to nourish your body.

Let's face it; change can be difficult, but not forever. Research studies show it takes approximately two to three weeks of repeated behavior to form a habit, so if you can just stick with your routine for a little while, it will get easier.

You've learned about the pro and cons of various elements of diets. Now it is time for you to implement what you've learned. Based upon the information that you've read, what modifications will you implement to improve your health? What is the best balance for you? Habits can be very hard to break, especially if you have lived with them all of your life. Don't let your habits and routines be a barrier. You can conquer unhealthy eating habits while developing a satisfying and healthy diet. Parts of your new diet may be very mentally challenging, but don't let anything get in the way of your victory. Everything feels funny at first, but don't stop at the funny feelings. If you wear anything long it enough it feels comfortable, so try it on.

Only you can decide what is best for you. It is obvious that you want to change. A more drastic change obviously will provide more drastic results, but how long will you be able to maintain drastic changes? Whatever modifications that you decide to implement in your diet, it is important that you maintain them, not only for weight loss, but for your health. A diet should not be an extreme measure to get you to your desired weight; rather a nutritional regimen that provides you with the nutrients and energy that you need to live your best life.

Although there are obstacles in the way of modifying your diet, there is nothing that you cannot achieve. Transitioning to a new diet can be tough; however, you can do it. Your stomach will adjust and it will be grateful to you.

While losing weight, be patient with yourself. Most likely you didn't put all the weight on in one week, one month, or even a year, so don't expect it to come off fast. One year can go by in the blink of an eye, so dedicate the effort to get the pounds off and it will be over before you know it.

We want the best for our family and friends, especially when we learn a new and better way, but eagerness can be a repellent; no good deed goes unpunished. Be the change that you want to see in your friends and family. Once they see the fruits of your efforts, they may be eager to learn your strategy.

Multiple lines of defense in the form of dietary knowledge, effort, and exercise is the best way to lose weight. Although losing weight may come at the compromise of a few indulgences, good health is a priceless gift that only you can give to yourself. Enjoying life today and tomorrow is the true reward. Hopefully you have gained some information that has better equipped you to find success in your journey to lose weight. Over time we may forget and lose focus. I hope that this book will be a reference for you to revisit to reinforce key concepts and a source of encouragement to keep you motivated. Believe in yourself, put your best efforts forth, and success will follow. Happy Living!

Appendix 1

103 Weight Management Tips and Strategies

I F IT SEEMS LIKE THERE ARE some tips and tricks to being healthy, there are. The following pages review some of the strategies mentioned throughout the book that may help you make better decisions and enhance your progress. Along your journey, you'll probably develop some strategies of your own.

1. Limit dairy
   + Fattening and loaded with saturated fat
2. Never eat second servings
   + Seconds increase the likelihood of overeating
   + Fill up on a piece of fruit, vegetables, or water
3. Eat beans and lentils
   + Good source of fiber, proteins, and nutrients
4. Eat dark greens
   + Good source of nutrients
   + The greener, the more nutrients
5. Reduce refined carbohydrates
   + High on calories + low on nutrients = empty calories
6. Always taste food before you add salt
   + Never sprinkle out of habit

7. Avoid skipping meals to lose weight
   + May slow your metabolism
8. Use a small plate
   + Helps reduce overeating
9. Eat slowly
   + Helps you eat less and recognize fullness
10. Fill up on plant products
    + Fewer calories and more nutrients
11. Pack your lunch
    + Don't be at the mercy of unhealthy food alternatives
12. Plan meals
    + Help ensure good meal choices
13. Expand your taste buds
    + Give foods multiple chances
    + You'll never know what you're missing unless you try it
14. Try new combinations of fruits and vegetables
    + Packed with nutrients to nourish your body
15. Limit saturated fat
    + Promotes heart disease and poor health
16. Eat lean meats
    + Less saturated fat
    + A good source of protein
17. Eat before you grocery shop
    + Helps avoid cravings
18. Shop with a list
    + Stay focused and away from temptations
    + If you don't buy it, you won't eat it
19. Eat before parties
    + Stay in control
    + Helps reduce uncontrollable snacking
20. Limit meat to the size of a deck of cards
    + Typical portions are oversized

✦ Too much meat may impede digestion

21. Eat fish once a week
 ✦ Good source of omega-3
22. Reduce or replace bread with veggies or fruit
 ✦ Most bread is refined with limited nutrients
23. Replace fries, potatoes, and rice with whole grains
 ✦ Good source of fiber
24. Eat sandwiches open-faced
 ✦ Reduce refined carbohydrates
25. Order smaller portions
 ✦ Appetizer, kiddy, luncheon, petite, salad, or halve it
26. Never supersize
 ✦ Opt for small portions
 ✦ Reduce excess calories
27. Request substitutes
 ✦ Make your meal healthier
28. Wrap your burger in a slice of lettuce
 ✦ Reduce refined carbs and increase nutrients
29. Wait before eating more
 ✦ 20 minutes may help your body recognize fullness
30. Sneak vegetable into all meals
 ✦ Spinach, eggplant, and squash blend seamlessly with many foods
31. Use nonstick cookware
 ✦ Requires less oil and butter to cook food
32. Use water or a mild vinegar instead of oil or butter to sauté food
 ✦ Less calories
33. Use healthy cooking styles
 ✦ Baked, grilled, roasted, and steamed
 ✦ Enhances flavors with fewer calories
34. Keep frozen vegetables available
 ✦ Healthy dinner option in minutes

35. Cook with olive oil
    + Fewer calories than butter
    + Add oil last to keep it healthy
36. Skip refined carbohydrates at breakfast
    + Low nutritional value
    + Eat fresh fruit
37. Select cereals with at least five grams of fiber
    + Watch out for excess sugar
    + Fiber is loaded with benefits
38. Add fruits and vegetables to every meal
    + At least five servings per day
39. Eat breakfast
    + Kick-start your metabolism
40. Eat a balanced diet
    + Nourish your body
41. Limit alcohol
    + Empty calories
    + Negative side effects
42. Eliminate fruit juice and soda
    + Empty calories
    + Limited or zero nutrients
43. Limit caffeine
    + Addictive
    + Reduce negative side effects
44. Drink water
    + Revitalize and cleanse body
45. Dilute juice with water
    + Reduce calories
46. Drink unsweetened tea
    + Good source of flavonoids
47. Make a smoothie with fruits and vegetables
    + Good source of nutrients

48. Dine at home
    + Make it healthy
49. Don't eat two to three hours before sleep
    + Rest and rejuvenate body
50. Don't eat after dinner
    + Start your nightly fast
51. Eat a small piece of what you crave
    + Kill the craving and move on
52. Sweeten with fruit
    + Fewer calories and side effects than natural and artificial sweeteners
53. Limit baked goods
    + Empty calories
    + Source of refined flour, sugar, and saturated fat
54. Replace chocolate with cocoa powder
    + Fewer calories and additives
55. Kick the sugar habit
    + Reduce calories and inflammation
56. Replace candy with fruit
    + Less calories and packed with nutrients
57. Reduce sauces
    + Source of additives, calories, and carbohydrates
58. Eat until you are 70% full
    + Helps improve digestion
59. Use mustard instead of mayo
    + Fewer calories
60. Use roasted garlic as mayonnaise
    + Fewer calories and more nutrients
61. Use aged and smoked cheeses like asiago and parmesan
    + Use less with strong flavors
62. Make your own dressings
    + Fewer calories

+ Avoid strong vinegars: white and cider
+ Add a little oil to reduce the acidic flavor of the vinegar
+ Use mild vinegars like balsamic, raspberry, rice, sherry, or wine

63. Skip buttering and oiling your bread
    + Each teaspoon has at least 100 calories
64. Flavor foods with spices and herbs versus salt and butter
    + More nutrients and less fat
65. Never give up
    + If at first you don't succeed, you're not alone
66. Find a support group
    + It can help you through the tough times
67. Commit for life
    + Continue after your reach your goal
68. Stay motivated
    + Strengthen your resolve
69. Watch for hidden sugars
    + Candy, canned food, drinks, food, and sauces
70. Don't eliminate all fat
    + Unsaturated and polyunsaturated fat are good in the right quantities
71. Figure out why and when you eat more
    + Helps improve your efforts
72. Don't get caught in the hype
    + Fad diets promise the moon and the stars and deliver neither
73. Carefully review labels
    + Know what you're eating
74. Keep a journal
    + Review what works and what doesn't
75. Weigh often
    + Catch pesky pounds fast
76. Go nuts
    + Good source of protein and fiber

77. Don't graze
    + May eat too much
78. Chew gum
    + Fewer calories than food
79. Buy one treat, instead of a box or bag
    + Reduce temptations and satisfy craving
80. Eat small snacks every couple of hours
    + Help reduce hunger and overeating
81. Stay busy
    + Any extra movement helps
82. Exercise
    + Maximizes your dieting efforts
83. Buy a digital scale
    + Every little bit lost can build motivation
84. Have realistic expectations
    + Unrealistic expectations can be demotivating
85. Find a good way to deal with stress
    + Stress can pack on the pounds
86. Focus on improving your health
    + Just losing weight is not enough
87. Strive for a healthy weight range
    + Easier to reach
    + Keeps motivation higher
88. Don't rely on quick fixes
    + Usually don't work
89. Bring your own food to festivities
    + Ensure you have good options
90. Avoid pumpernickel and rye
    + Are not whole grain.
    + May be darkened with molasses
91. Eat brown rice instead of white rice
    + Healthier with almost three times the amount of fiber

92. Avoid allergens
    + Promotes inflammation
    + Reduces body's functioning
93. Avoid packaged food
    + Too many chemicals and refined carbohydrates
94. Avoid saturated and trans-fats
    + Select mono or unsaturated fats
95. Avoid artificial flavors
    + Fresh is best
96. Avoid preservatives
    + Eat fresh food as much as possible
97. Avoid MSG
    + Causes side effects
98. Avoid artificial sweeteners
    + Excessive chemicals and side effects
99. Carefully consider all pills
    + Negative side effects
100. Get enough sleep
    + Sleep improves the body's functioning
101. Reduce the stress
    + Too much stress is detrimental to the body
102. Get the facts about your meal
    + Ask the waiter
    + Review the nutrition labels
103. Reaffirm your goals daily
    + Post goals prominently

Appendix

Action Plan

2

N OW THAT YOU HAVE READ the book, what are some of the foods and drinks that you will reduce to unburden your body? What are some of the foods that you will add to nourish your body?

Granted, what you eat may change on a daily basis, but many of us are creatures of habit and our meals may have a familiar pattern. It is important to consider the foods and beverages that make up your diet and how they affect your health.

Example:

	Current Diet		Your Optimum Diet	
	Food	**Drink**	**Food**	**Drink**
Breakfast	Cereals	Coffee	Fruits and whole grains	Green tea
Snack	Chips	Soda	Fruits	Water
Lunch	Burgers, fries	Juice	Vegetables	Water w/ fruit
Snack	Candy bars	Soda	Fruits	Water
Dinner	Refined carbs & meat	Juice	Meats and veggies	Tea

	Current Diet		Your Optimum Diet	
	Food	**Drink**	**Food**	**Drink**
Breakfast				
Snack				
Lunch				
Snack				
Dinner				

Appendix 3

Quiz I: Find the Evil

IDENTIFY EVERYTHING THAT may negatively impact your health for the following items.

Example:

1. Donuts—refined flour
2. Chips
3. Soda
4. Fruit juice
5. Bread
6. 16 oz. porterhouse steak
7. Barbecue chicken
8. Salad with dressing
9. Meat loaf with gravy
10. Fish
11. Restaurant entrees
12. Fried food
13. Pasta
14. Cooked food
15. Sports drinks
16. Hamburgers
17. French fries
18. Ice cream
19. Candy
20. Artificial sweeteners

Answers to Quiz I: Find the Evil

While this list attempts to be exhaustive, there still may be additional good answers. The point of this exercise is to get you critically thinking about everything that you eat. If you identified at least one negative factor for each food you're off to a great start.

1. Donuts
    + Refined carbohydrates, fried in oil, and glazed with sugar
2. Chips
    + Refined carbohydrates, fried in oil, and doused with artificial flavors
3. Soda
    + Liquid sugar filled with artificial flavoring, caffeine, phosphoric acid, and natural or artificial sweeteners
4. Fruit juice
    + Artificial flavoring, preservatives, and sugar
5. Bread
    + Additives, preservatives, refined carbohydrates, and sugar
6. 16 oz. porterhouse steak
    + Antibiotics, hormones, pesticides, promotes acidic conditions in the body, saturated fat, and too much for one serving
7. Barbecue chicken
    + Artificial flavors, heterocyclic amines from grilling, and sugar
8. Salad with dressing
    + Dressing may have extra carbohydrates, oil, and sugar
    + Iceberg lettuce has limited nutrients
9. Meat loaf with gravy
    + Antibiotics, bread crumbs—refined carbohydrates, hormones, pesticides, saturated fat, and sugar
10. Fish
    + Beware of water contaminates like PCB and mercury

11. Restaurant entrees
    + Varies: excess calories and large serving sizes
12. Fried food
    + Bread crumbs, excess calories, saturated fats, and trans-fats
13. Pasta
    + Refined carbohydrates and fatty sauces
14. Cooked food
    + Limited nutrients
    + Negative by-products of cooking
15. Sports drinks
    + Extra sugar and preservatives
16. Hamburgers
    + Antibiotics, extra condiments, hormones, pesticides, and saturated fat
17. French fries
    + Acrylamides, excess salt, and saturated or trans-fat
18. Ice cream
    + Same dangers as beef: antibiotics, hormones, pesticides, and saturated fat
19. Candy
    + Artificial flavors, chemicals, and sugar
20. Artificial sweeteners
    + Chemicals and toxins

Appendix 4

Quiz II: Make It Better

How can you make each item better for you? The items listed are everyday items that you may come into contact with at one point or another. Critically think about how you can improve your meal.

1. Donuts
2. Chips
3. Soda
4. Fruit juice
5. Bread
6. 16 oz. porterhouse steak
7. Barbecue chicken
8. Salad with dressing
9. Meat loaf with gravy
10. Fish
11. Restaurant entrees
12. Fried food
13. Pasta
14. Cooked food
15. Sports drinks
16. Hamburgers
17. French fries
18. Ice cream
19. Candy
20. Artificial sweeteners

Answers to Quiz II: Make It Better

Same concept as the last quiz. The point is to help you think critically about how you can improve your meal. If you identify at least one thing for each number you're doing great.

1. Donuts
    + Select whole grain or plain donuts
2. Chips
    + Eat baked chips
3. Soda
    + Enjoy a small size
    + Drink organic soda
4. Fruit juice
    + Dilute with water
    + Juice fruits or vegetables
5. Bread
    + Select whole grain bread
6. 16 oz. porterhouse steak
    + Reduce the portion size, share, or save it for later
7. Barbecue chicken
    + Bake in oven
    + Bake with herbs
    + Reduce or eliminate sauce
8. Salad with dressing
    + Make a vinaigrette
    + Eat romaine lettuce
9. Meat loaf with gravy
    + Eat organic meat
    + Lose the gravy
    + Add veggies
10. Fish
    + Eat a low contaminated fish once per week

11. Restaurant entrees
   + Request healthy options
   + Reduce portion size
12. Fried food
   + Bake or sauté instead
13. Pasta
   + Select whole grain pasta
   + Add veggies
14. Cooked food
   + Add raw fruits and lightly steamed vegetables
15. Sports drinks
   + Drink water
16. Hamburgers
   + Lean, open-faced, limited condiments, and add extra veggies
17. French fries
   + Eat baked sweet potato fries
18. Ice cream
   + Blend frozen fruit
19. Candy
   + Eat dried fruit or nuts
20. Artificial sweeteners
   + Sweeten with fruit

Appendix 5
Shopping List

WHILE THIS LIST IS not exhaustive, these are some great foods to stock your cupboard with on a weekly basis to help promote your weight loss and health improvement efforts

Grains
Brown rice
Cereal ≥ 5 grams
   of fiber
Steel cut oatmeal
Whole wheat pitas
Whole wheat pasta
Whole wheat bread
Whole wheat
tortillas

Cans/Jars
Corn
Fruit
Beans

Tomatoes
Tomato sauce

Nuts
Walnuts
Almonds
Hazelnuts

Condiments
Salt
Pepper
Olive oil
Fresh garlic
Balsamic vinegar

Beverages
Tea
Water

Refrigerated Items
Eggs
Plain yogurt

Meat
Fish
Lean meat

Frozen Food
Fruits
Vegetables

Produce

Lime	Tomato	Raspberries
Garlic	Onions	Blueberries
Plums	Avocado	blackberries
Lemon	Bananas	sweet potatoes
Carrots	Eggplant	bell peppers
Apples	Asparagus	green beans
	Fresh herbs	dark green lettuces

Appendix 6

Journal

    Can you remember every bite and sip that you took every day last week? Most of us can't accurately remember everything that we ate yesterday that is why keeping a journal is so important. Every single bite you take has the ability to affect your weight loss, so it is crucial to keep track of everything you eat and drink. The information that you record in your journal may help you learn what catapults and what diminishes your weight loss. Your journal is strictly for you and every bite counts; so record accurately.

Journal						
Date		Weight				
Ate five fruits/veggies		Hours of sleep				
Mood		Workout	Y / N	How long?		

Meal	Time	
Breakfast		
Drink		
Other		
Snack		
Drink		
Other		
Lunch		
Drink		
Other		
Snack		
Drink		
Other		
Dinner		
Drink		
Other		

References

Allan, B. & Lutz, W. (2000). *Life without bread: How a low-carbohydrate diet can save your life.* New York: McGraw Hill.

American Heart Association (2009). Fat. Retrieved July 25, 2009 from http://www.americanheart.org/presenter. jhtml?identifier=4582

American Heart Association (n.d.). Know Your Fats. Retrieved July 25, from http://www.americanheart.org/presenter. jhtml?identifier=532

American Heart Association. (n.d.). LDL and HDL Cholesterol: What's Bad and What's Good? Retrieved July 25, 2009 from http://www.americanheart.org/presenter.jhtml?identifier=180

Batmanghelidj, F. (2003). *Water: for health, for healing, for life: You're not sick, you're thirsty!* New York: Warner Books.

Beale, L. & Clark, J. (2005). *The complete idiot's guide to: Glycemic index weight loss.* New York: Penguin Books.

Bennett, C. & Sinatra, S. (2007). *Sugar shock!* New York: Berkeley Books.

Blaylock, R. (1997). *Excitotoxins: The taste that kills.* Santa Fe, NM: Health Press.

Boutenko, V. (2007). *12 steps to raw foods: How to end your dependency on cooked food.* (Rev. ed.). Berkeley: North Atlantic Books.

Bridson, K. (2006). *The secrets of skinny chicks: How to feel great in your favorite jeans—when it doesn't come naturally.* New York: McGraw Hill.

Center for Disease Control (n.d.). *Obesity: Halting the Epidemic by Making Health Easier At A Glance 2009.* Retrieved July 30, 2009, from http://www.cdc.gov/NCCdphp/publications/AAG/obesity.htm

Challem, J. (2003). *The inflammation syndrome: The complete nutritional program to prevent and reverse heart disease, arthritis, diabetes, allergies, and asthma.* Hoboken, NJ: John Wiley & Sons, Inc.

Campbell, T. Colin, & Campbell, Thomas M. (2006). *The China study: the most comprehensive study of nutrition ever conducted and the startling implications for diet, weight loss and long-term health.* Dallas, TX: Benbella Books

Coghill, T. (2008, March 14). *Fasting and stomach size.* Retrieved June 22, 2009 from http://www.fasting.ws/juice-fasting/fasting-questions/fasting-shrink-stomach.

Downer, J. (n.d.). *How to become a competitive eater.* Retrieved June 22, 2009, from http://www.ehow.com/how_214 2152_become-competitive-eater.html

Drummond, K. (n.d.). *Sugar Fuels Tumor Growth, Says Major New Study.* Retrieved February 9, 2010, from http://www.aolnews.com/health/article/study-in-singapore-links-sugary-soft-drinks-and-pancreatic-cancer/19348936?icid=main|hp-laptop|dl1|link3|http%3A%2F%2Fwww.aolnews.com%2Fhealth%2Farticle%2Fstudy-in-singapore-links-sugary-soft-drinks-and-pancreatic-cancer%2F19348936

EHealth MD. (n.d.). *Fiber: Its Importance In Your Diet.* Retrieved July 30, 2009, from http://www.ehealthmd.com/library/fiber/FIB_whatis.html

EPA (n.d.). *Polychlorinated Biphenyls (PCBs) Update: Impact on Fish Advisories.* Retrieved July 25, 2009, from http://www.epa.gov/waterscience/fish/files/pcbs.pdf

Essortment (n.d.). *Nutritional benefits of beans.* Retrieved January 10, 2010, from http://www.essortment.com/all/benefitsofbean_rbdb.htm

Fife, B. (2001). *The detox book: how to detoxify your body to improve your health, stop disease and reverse aging.* (Rev. 2nd ed.). Colorado Springs, CO: Piccadilly Book, Ltd.

Food Allergy & Anaphylaxis Network (n.d.). Retrieved July 30, 2009, from http://www.foodallergy.org/

Foods for life (n.d.). *Plant based sources of vegan & vegetarian Docosahexaenoic acid—DHA and Eicosapentaenoic acid EPA & Essential Fats.* Retrieved July 24, 2009, from http://www.vegetarian-dha-epa.co.uk/

Food Standards Agency (n.d.). *Organic Food.* Retrieved July 31, 2009, from http://www.food.gov.uk/foodindustry/farmingfood/organicfood/

Fuhrman, J. (2003). *Eat to live: The revolutionary formula for fast and sustained weight loss.* New York: Little, Brown and Company.

Freedman, R. & Barnes, K. (2005). *Skinny bitch.* Philadelphia: Running Press.

Galland, L. (2005). *The fat resistance diet.* New York: Broadway Books.

Gittleman, A. (2002). *The fat flush plan.* New York: McGraw Hill.

Global Healing Center (n.d.). *All Vitamins Are Not Created Equal.* Retrieved July 31, 2009, from http://www.globalhealingcenter.com/all-vitamins-are-not-created-equal.html

Hackett, J. (n.d.) *Top 7 Types of Vegetarians.* About. Retrieved June 22, 2010, from http://vegetarian.about.com/od/vegetarianvegan101/tp/TypesofVeg.htm

Hatch, A. (2009, August 13). *Organic Foods May Not Be Healthier.* Parent Dish. Retrieved September 3,

2009, from http://www.parentdish.com/2009/08/13/organic-foods-may-not-be-healthier-report-says

Hawthorne, F. (2005). *Inside of the FDA: The business and politics behind the drugs we take and the food that we eat.* Hoboken, NJ: John Wiley & Sons, Inc.

Healing Daily (n.d.). *Is soy safe?* Retrieved October 28, 2009, from http://www.healingdaily.com/detoxification-diet/soy.htm

Isaacs, S. (2007). *Hormonal Balance: Understanding hormones, weight, and your metabolism.* Boulder: Bull Publishing Company.

Janeway, J. Sparks, K., & Baker, R. (2007). *The real skinny on weight loss surgery: An indispensable guide of way you can really expect!* (2nd ed.). Onondaga, MI: Little Victories Press.

Johnson, S. (2009, January 2). *The Benefits Of Beans: 9 Reasons Why YOU Should Eat Beans. Bliss Plan.* Retrieved Jan. 9th 2010, from http://www.blissplan.com/wellness-fitness/the-benefits-of-beans-9-reasons-why-you-should-eat-beans

Kirby, J. (2004). *Dieting for dummies.* (2nd ed.). Hoboken, NJ: Wiley Publishing, Inc.

Kuhn, C., Swartzwelder, S., & Wilson, W. (2008) *Buzzed: The straight facts about the most used and abused drugs from alcohol to ecstasy.* (Rev. 3rd ed.). New York: W. W. Norton & Company.

Kurian, M., Thompson, B., & Davidson, B. (2005). *Weight loss surgery for dummies.* Indianapolis: Wiley Publishing, Inc. Lieberman, S. & Segall, L. (2007). *The gluten connection: How gluten sensitivity may be sabotaging your health- and what you can do to take control now.* New York: Rodale.

Mayo Clinic (n.d.). *Supplements: What to know before you buy.* Retrieved June 22, 2009, from http://mayoclinic.com/health/herbalsupplements/SA00044/NSECTIONGROUP=2

Mercola, J. & Pearsall, K. (2006). *Sweet deception: Why Splenda®, Nutrasweet®, and the FDA may be hazardous to your health.* Nashville, TN: Thomas Nelson, Inc.

Meyerowitz, S. (2002) *Juice fasting and detoxification.* (6th ed.). Summerton, TN: Book Publishing Company.

Mindell, E. & Mundis, H. (2004). *Earl Mindell's new vitamin bible* (Rev. ed.). New York: Warner Books

Murray, M. (1998). *The complete book of juicing.* (2nd ed.). New York: Three River Press.

National Coalition on Health Care. (n.d.) *Health Insurance Cost.* Retrieved June 23, 2009, from http://www.nchc.org/facts/cost. shtml

National Health and Nutrition Examination Survey (2004). Retrieved August 1, 2009, from http://www.cdc.gov/nchs/ nhanes.htm

National Institute of Diabetes and Digestive and Kidney Disease (n.d.). *Statistics related to overweight and obesity.* Retrieved June 14, 2008, from http://win.niddk.nih.gov/statistics/

National Institute of Health (n.d.). Retrieved July 20, 2009, from http://www.nih.gov/

New England Journal of Medicine (n.d.). *Comparison of Weight-Loss Diets with Different Compositions of Fat, Protein, and Carbohydrates.* Retrieved July 31, 2009, from http://www.nejm. org/doi/full/10.1056/NEJMoa0804748

Ni, M. (2006). *Secrets of longevity: Hundreds of ways to live to be 100.* San Francisco: Chronicle Book.

World Health Organization (n.d.). *Obesity and overweight.* Retrieved July 25, 2009, from http://www.who.int/ mediacentre/factsheets/fs311/en/index.html

Oski, F. (1996). *Don't drink your milk! New frightening medical facts about the world's most overrated nutrient.* Brushton: Teach Services, Inc.

Pitchford, P. (2002). *Healing with whole foods: Asian traditions and modern nutrition.* (Rev. 3rd ed.). Berkeley, CA: North Atlantic Books.

Porter, J. (2004). *The hip chick's guide to macrobiotics: A philosophy for achieving a radiant mind and fabulous body.* New York: Avery.

Rinzler, C (2006). *Nutrition for dummies.* (4th ed.). Hoboken: Wiley Publishing.

Roizen, M. & Oz, M. (2006). *You: On a diet; The owner's manual for waist management.* New York: Free Press.

Schlosser, E. (2002), *Fast food nation: the dark side of the all-American meal.* New York: Harper Perennial.

Science Daily (2010, January 6). *Restaurant and Packaged Foods Can Have More Calories Than Nutrition Labeling Indicates.* Retrieved March 2, 2010, from http://www.sciencedaily.com/releases/2010/01/100105100021.htm

Steward, H., Andrews, S., Morrison, B., & Balart, L. (2003). *The New Sugar Busters! Cut sugar to trim fat.* New York: Ballantine Books.

Stöppler, C. & Marks, J. W. (n.d.). *Medications and Drugs.* Retrieved January 9, 2010, from http://www.medicinenet.com/oral_contraceptives_birth_control_pills/page2.htm

Sweet, M. (2010, February 16). *What's the difference between omega-3's, 6's and 9's? Women to Women.* Retrieved June 28, 2010, from http://www.womentowomen.com/healthynutrition/differencebetweenomega369.aspx

UHealthy (n.d.). *Grain-Fed versus Grass-Fed Animal Products.* Retrieved September 3, 2009, from http://www.nwhealth.edu/healthyU/eatWell/grassfed.html

Wiki (n.d.). *What is pasteurization?* Retrieved July 24, 2009, from http://wiki.answers.com/Q/What_is_pasteurization

Wikipedia. (n.d.). *Dietary fiber.* Retrieved August 1, 2009, from http://en.wikipedia.org/wiki/Dietary_fiber

Wikipedia (n.d.). *Nosocomial infection.* Retrieved June 24, 2009, from http://en.wikipedia.org/wiki/Nosocomial_infection

Wisegeek (n.d.). What is Gluten? Retrieved July 30, 2009, from http://www.wisegeek.com/what-is-gluten.htm

Wisegeek (n.d.). *What Is Nut Milk?* Retrieved July 29, 2009 from http://www.wisegeek.com/what-is-nut-milk.htm

Wisegeek (n.d.). *What is Rice Milk?* Retrieved July 29, 2009 from http://www.wisegeek.com/what-is-rice-milk.htm

Wisegeek (n.d.). *What is Soy Milk?* Retrieved July 30, 2009 from http://www.wisegeek.com/what-is-soy-milk.htm

Willett, W. (2001). *Eat, drink, and be healthy: The Harvard Medical school guide to healthy eating.* New York: Free Press.

World's Healthiest Foods. (n.d.). *Food Sensitivities.* Retrieved April 21, 2010, from http://www.whfoods.com/genpage.php?tname=faq&dbid=30

Wrong Diagnosis (n.d.). *How Common is Misdiagnosis?* Retrieved June 24, 2009 from http://www.wrongdiagnosis.com/intro/common.htm

Index

Quick Order Form

Fax orders: 1-914-835-0398

Telephone orders: Call 1-800-431-1579. Please have your credit card ready.

E-mail orders: orders@bookch.com

Postal orders: BCH Fulfillment & Distribution, 46 Purdy Street, Harrison, New York 10528

Online: www.devalentino.com (Click Orders)

Please send *How to Lose Weight in the Real World: Why Other Diets Suck and You're Not Losing Weight.* I understand that I may return it for a full refund-for any reason.

Name: _____

Address: _____

City: _____

State: _____ Zip: _____

Telephone: ( ) _____

E-mail _____

Credit Card No. _____

Card Exp. _____

Signature: _____

Shipping: US: $4. Add $2 for each additional book.
International: $9. Add $5 for each additional book.

Book $19.95 x _____ = _____

Shipping _____

Total _____

Quick Order Form

Fax orders: 1-914-835-0398

Telephone orders: Call 1-800-431-1579. Please have your credit card ready.

E-mail orders: orders@bookch.com

Postal orders: BCH Fulfillment & Distribution, 46 Purdy Street, Harrison, New York 10528

Online: www.devalentino.com (Click Orders)

Please send *How to Lose Weight in the Real World: Why Other Diets Suck and You're Not Losing Weight.* I understand that I may return it for a full refund-for any reason.

Name: _____

Address: _____

City: _____

State: _____ Zip: _____

Telephone: (_____) _____

E-mail _____

Credit Card No. _____

Card Exp. _____

Signature: _____

Shipping: US: $4. Add $2 for each additional book.

International: $9. Add $5 for each additional book.

Book $19.95 x _____ = _____

Shipping _____

Total _____